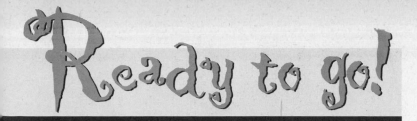

IDEAS FOR
PSHE

KS2

P4 to 7

D0239392

AUTHOR
Ingrid Oliver

DESIGNER
David Hurley

EDITOR
Clare Gallaher

ILLUSTRATIONS
Debbie Clark

ASSISTANT EDITOR
Roanne Davis

COVER ARTWORK
Ian Murray

SERIES DESIGNER
Anna Oliwa

Text © 2000 Ingrid Oliver
© 2000 Scholastic Ltd

Designed using Adobe Pagemaker
Published by Scholastic Ltd, Villiers House, Clarendon
Avenue, Leamington Spa, Warwickshire CV32 5PR
Printed by Bell & Bain Ltd, Glasgow

34567890 123456789

British Library Cataloguing-in-Publication Data
A catalogue record for this book is available from the
British Library.

ISBN 0-439-01670-3

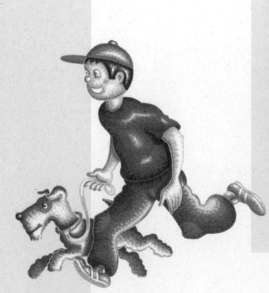

The right of Ingrid Oliver to be identified as the author
of this work has been asserted by her in accordance
with the Copyright, Designs and Patents Act 1988.

All rights reserved. This book is sold subject to the
condition that it shall not, by way of trade or otherwise,
be lent, hired out or otherwise circulated without the
publisher's prior consent in any form of binding or cover
other than that in which it is published and without a
similar condition, including this condition, being imposed
upon the subsequent purchaser.

No part of this publication may be reproduced, stored
in a retrieval system, or transmitted, in any form or by
any means, electronic, mechanical, photocopying,
recording or otherwise, without the prior permission
of the publisher. This book remains copyright, although
permission is granted to copy those pages marked
'Photocopiables' for classroom distribution and use
only in the school which has purchased the book and
in accordance with the CLA licensing agreement.
Photocopying permission is given only for purchasers
and not for borrowers of books from any lending
service.

Contents

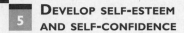
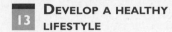

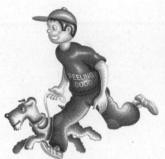

Introduction

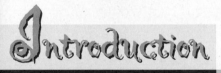

Personal, social and health education has been recognized as fundamental in enabling children to take increasing responsibility for their own learning, and hence to maximize their potential. This style of education has been found to help children cope with social pressure affecting their learning, so raising standards of academic achievement, which in itself enhances their self-esteem and their personal health and well-being.

ABOUT THIS BOOK

Many of the types of activities in this book will be familiar to teachers. However, to facilitate curriculum planning they are arranged in a framework which is compatible with the Government guidelines for Personal, Social and Health Education (PSHE) and Citizenship for Key Stages 1 and 2 (*Preparing Young People for Adult Life*, DfEE, May 1999).

The activities will support teaching towards the four given government objectives which are to help pupils to:

■ develop self-esteem, confidence, independence and responsibility, and make the most of their abilities
■ play an active role as future citizens
■ develop a healthy lifestyle and keep themselves and others safe
■ develop effective and fulfilling relationships and learn to respect the differences between people.

Information on how to organize each activity is provided in such a way that teachers can easily adapt it to the needs of children of different abilities. The particular skills to be developed are linked to the National Standards for Key Skills, with an easy-check skills index. Suggestions are given throughout for follow-up work. The activities are given within the framework of 'Outcomes of personal and social development' suggested by the Calouste Gulbenkian Foundation's PASSPORT project. The following eight sections have been adapted from this. They provide opportunities to enable children to:

- develop self-esteem and self-confidence
- develop a healthy lifestyle
- learn to keep themselves and others safe
- develop effective and satisfying relationships
- learn to respect the differences between people
- develop independence and responsibility
- learn to become good citizens
- make the most of their abilities.

IDEAS FOR PSHE KEY STAGE I (PI TO 3)

The activities in this lead-in book are arranged under the same headings as in *Ideas for PSHE Key Stage 2 (P4 to 7)*, and provide for a built-in progression. Some activities are directly linked, so you are able to select those most appropriate for the abilities and interests of your classes.

At both stages, the activities can be integrated into a variety of curriculum areas, including healthy schools, citizenship or world of work programmes.

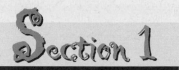
DEVELOP SELF-ESTEEM AND SELF-CONFIDENCE

The activities in this section focus on children:
■ expressing positive qualities about themselves and others
■ recognizing feelings in different situations and what might cause them, and managing them.
■ knowing personal likes and dislikes
■ expressing feelings in different ways and understanding their impact on others.

BODY LANGUAGE

RESOURCES AND CLASSROOM ORGANIZATION

You will need: a copy of photocopiable page 12 (enlarged if possible) for each child, and an enlarged copy cut up into the six characters and pasted on six large pieces of paper (one character at the top of each sheet), displayed on the walls of the classroom; writing materials.

Children work in groups, then as a class.

WHAT TO DO

Introduce the topic of how animals communicate with one another by asking the children to think about pets – dogs and cats in particular. *How can we tell if a dog is happy, excited, sad or frightened?* (Posture, tail wagging and so on.). Pets can 'talk' without using words. We can guess what they're feeling by looking at their whole body – we call this 'body language'. *Do you think humans communicate in this way?*

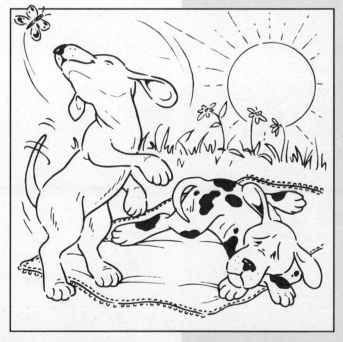

Divide the class into six groups and number them 1 to 6. Explain that they are going to look closely at human 'body language' and try to work out what each of six characters are feeling. Give everyone a copy of photocopiable page 12 and ask each child to decide what they think each person is feeling, and to take turns to share their ideas with their group.

All the children should then try to write two or three words describing the feelings under each character. The characters portray 1. Misery, 2. Joy, 3. Envy, 4. Anger, 5. Anxiety, 6. Frustration. Move round the groups, helping with the interpretations.

Next, ask each group to say what words they have chosen for the possible feelings (emotions) of one of the characters (the character who has the same number as the group). List these on the relevant large sheet displayed on the classroom wall. Can other groups add any suggestions? Discuss the results. The interpretations may well overlap, demonstrating that body language can be tricky to interpret – so when trying to discover how someone feels it might also help if we ask, 'How are you feeling?'

Now ask each group to discuss *one* way in which the character that they have been allocated might help himself (or herself) to 'manage' the feeling. For example, if 'angry', character 4 could use a punchbag, not a person, and talk to a friend. Ask a volunteer from each group to write these ideas at the bottom of the relevant large sheet displayed on the wall.

OBJECTIVES

To enable children to:
■ explore non-verbal communication (body language)
■ develop a vocabulary for expressing emotions
■ begin to understand how to cope with different emotions.

CROSS-CURRICULAR LINKS

ENGLISH

Responding appropriately to others; predicting outcomes; discussing; drama.

ART

Appreciating the different ways in which ideas, feelings and meanings are communicated in visual form.

Once all six are completed, suggest that children walk around the room, reading the ideas about how to cope with the emotion, and adding any ideas of their own if they wish.

Discuss the 'managing emotions' ideas with the whole class, and add others if appropriate. Ask the class to reflect on what they have learned during the lesson. How might they be able to make use of this learning in the future?

NOW OR LATER

■ This work particularly lends itself to mime and role-play. Groups could prepare (a) a single character 'pose', to be interpreted by the rest of the class, and (b) a two-person 'pose' where the others have to interpret what has happened and what the relationship is between the two. More able children might create a mime scene using several characters, interacting, but silent, to be discussed and interpreted by the rest of the class.

■ Examples of works of art, pictures and sculptures showing body postures could be made into a display and appropriate children's work in art sessions added to these.

■ All this work could be developed for presentation at assemblies or open days.

WITH THE COMPLIMENTS OF THE CLASS

OBJECTIVES
To enable children to:
■ express positive qualities about themselves and others
■ have the self-confidence to accept praise
■ develop the interpersonal skill of encouraging others and the cognitive skills of reflecting and evaluating
■ generate a positive, supportive atmosphere in the classroom.

CROSS-CURRICULAR LINKS
ENGLISH
Responding appropriately to others; developing speaking and listening skills; increasing vocabulary.

RESOURCES AND CLASSROOM ORGANIZATION
You will need: a chalkboard/whiteboard; a large sheet of paper for each child (for example, two sheets of A4 fixed end to end), divided into as many sections as there are pupils; a clipboard or book for each child to rest the paper on; writing materials.

Children work as a class or half class, then as individuals and finish with a class discussion. In this activity, papers are passed around the class (as in the game 'Consequences') and you will need to plan a systematic method of passing them around so that everyone writes on every sheet. (An easy way to do this might be to sit in one large circle, facing outwards for confidentiality!)

WHAT TO DO
Start with a discussion about the ways in which we can praise people by complimenting them on their good qualities. Write examples on the board. These might be: a person having 'a nice smile', being 'cheerful, enthusiastic, caring', or being helpful, such as 'holding the door open for me' and so on . Try to get a good selection, so that each child will be able to choose something suitable for everyone else when they play the following 'game'.

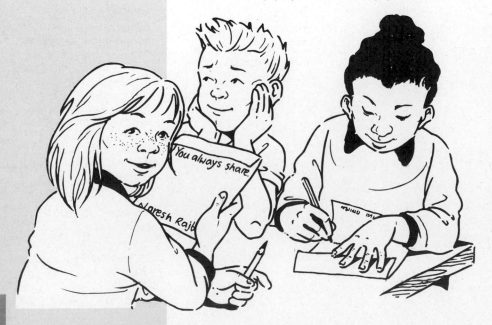

Explain that you are going to give each child a sheet of paper for them to write their own name clearly at the *bottom*. When everyone has done this, they all pass their sheet clockwise to the person on their *right*. Next they write a compliment (anonymously) for the child whose name appears at the bottom of the sheet. The compliment is written at the *top* of the sheet and then the sheet is folded down to hide the writing before passing the sheet on. No peeping allowed! Let them have a short time to think of what to write before writing.

When everyone has written on every sheet, each one is passed to the child whose name appears at the bottom. Everyone reads their own sheet. Each child now reads out some comments they have chosen from the sheet. A friend could do this for them if they are too embarrassed! The child thanks the class for their compliments, and gets a round of applause.

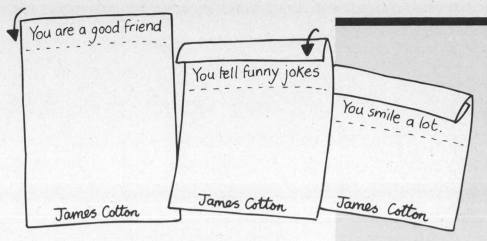

When everyone has had their turn, finish by discussing with the class what they have discovered:

■ *What does it feel like to receive compliments?* (Hopefully they will conclude that it feels good!)
■ *So why is it important to praise people?* (It gives them encouragement, raises their self-esteem and so on.)
■ *What is it like to give a compliment? Did it make you think of something good about someone that you hadn't appreciated before?*
■ *Should everyone be valued? Is it helpful to emphasize the good qualities in everyone?*
■ *What would it be like if we never received any praise from anyone?*

NOW OR LATER

■ Each child could put their compliments sheet in a file, or inside their desk lid, to look at from time to time, or they could be mounted and displayed if appropriate.
■ Ask the children to write a summary of what they have learned during the session (see the questions above).
■ The class could make a pledge to try to compliment each other more often. Display a 'compliment pledge' on the wall.

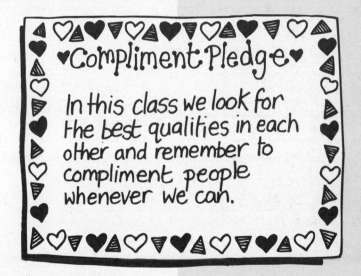

BE A GOOD LISTENER

RESOURCES AND CLASSROOM ORGANIZATION

You will need: a jotter or notebook for each child; class sheets of large paper headed: 'When we both talked at once we felt…' and, 'When we listened to each other we felt…'; writing materials.

Children work in pairs for most of the activity.

WHAT TO DO

Introduce the activity by explaining to the class that people may not always be good at really listening when someone is talking to them. Also, when people talk to us we may not always respond to them in a way they find helpful. Therefore they are going to do some research on these two situations in the following way.

Ask the children to work in pairs. Explain that they are going to tell their partner about any topic that really interests them, such as pets, holidays, clubs, sports activities, books they have read, TV programmes, and so on. Give them a few moments to think about a topic.

Now ask both children to talk at the same time, and to try hard to keep going for three minutes or more. You can time them if you wish, or some children might like to time themselves.

OBJECTIVES

To enable children to:
■ develop the interpersonal skill of encouraging others
■ develop the cognitive skills of reflecting and evaluating
■ recognize feelings in different situations
■ reflect on the strengths and weaknesses of their listening skills
■ give and receive positive feedback
■ develop empathy skills.

CROSS-CURRICULAR LINKS

ENGLISH

Speaking and listening skills; extended writing; drama.

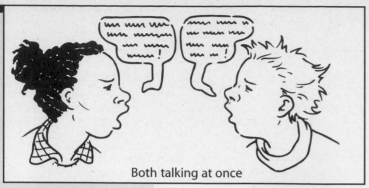

Both talking at once

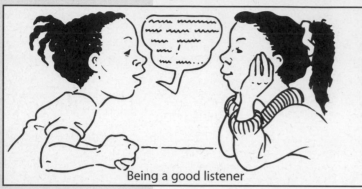

Being a good listener

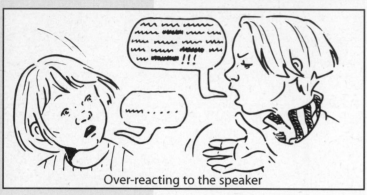

Over-reacting to the speaker

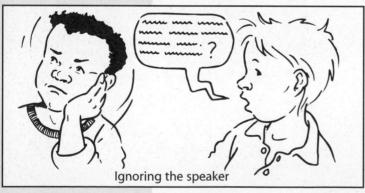

Ignoring the speaker

Next, ask them to take it in turns to speak about the same topic, and this time the listener must try to listen well – so discuss what this might mean. (Concentrating, thinking about the speaker's feelings, giving short feedback to support the speaker, such as 'Do you?', 'That's interesting' or 'How do you feel about that?' Body language is important too – looking interested, perhaps nodding and looking into someone's eyes when they are talking to you.)

If you want an extra level of sophistication here, add a second round of conversation. Suggest that one of the pair does not respond at all when being talked to (he or she looks away, doesn't reply and so on) or alternatively over-reacts by responding loudly and excitedly and 'taking over' from the speaker.

Ask the children to discuss what happened and how they felt on each occasion, and jot down their findings.

■ *What was it like when you both spoke at once? How did you feel?* (Frustrated, angry, disempowered.)

■ *What was it like to be really listened to?* (It felt good – it made me feel important and reassured. I enjoyed the feeling of liking my friend.)

■ (If appropriate) *What was it like when someone did not respond to you, or responded too much?* (I felt hurt, rejected, sad, unimportant, ignored, discounted, put down, taken over, overwhelmed, flattened.)

The pair could also consider what they have found out about their partner and if they have anything in common which they did not realize before.

Now ask the pairs to join up to make fours, and to compare their notes on each of the situations. Ask one person from each quartet to write the group's most important feelings on the appropriate class sheets.

Finally, discuss the results and ask the class to reflect on the activity and what they have learned from it. How will they be able to use this knowledge in the future?

NOW OR LATER

■ Children could write down how they felt about the activity and what they have learned. Were they good listeners before? How might they improve their listening in everyday life?

■ Pairs could now work on their activities to produce a mini drama which demonstrates to people what a good listener is and why it is important to be a good listener.

■ Ask the children to write a story that starts with someone trying to tell somebody something. The story is given two possible endings – one where the speaker is *not* listened to and the consequences, and the other where the speaker *is* listened to and the consequences. (For example, the stories could start with 'I think I might have discovered some buried treasure' or 'I've just seen your dog and he looked as if he'd found something interesting'.)

LOOKING AHEAD – HOPES AND FEARS

RESOURCES AND CLASSROOM ORGANIZATION

You will need: a large sheet of paper for each small group; board or flip chart; writing and drawing materials.

Children work in groups, then as a class.

WHAT TO DO

Introduce the activity by suggesting that everyone has hopes and fears now and for the future. Explain that the children are going to explore this by considering what an invented character, a boy or girl of their age, might be worried about. (By using this method children can safely reveal any concerns through the characters, thus protecting confidentiality.)

Divide the class into small groups and ask each group to invent and name a boy or girl, and then discuss and list his or her possible worries (including any imaginary ones such as being kidnapped by aliens!). If time allows, let the children draw their characters as well.

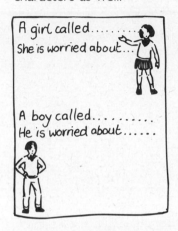

A girl called ....
She is worried about ...

A boy called ....
He is worried about ......

Once the groups have decided on their character, and discussed and listed their worries, ask them to take it in turns to introduce their character and his or her worries to the rest of the class. The class should then discuss possible solutions to the worries.

List key worries on the board, together with possible solutions in each case, with an emphasis on who would be able to help. For older Key Stage 2 children these often include:

■ starting secondary school
(Possible solutions: organize a school visit to express concerns; identify friends with whom the person can go to school; give reassurance that everyone finds it strange at first.) See also 'Expectations of secondary school' on page 48.

■ getting spots/starting periods/other concerns about puberty
(Possible solutions: the school plans for lessons/television programmes covering these changes; the person talks to a parent/teacher/school nurse/doctor/friend; obtains books from the local or school library; reads leaflets for ten-year-olds from commercial organizations or charities such as Brook.)

■ teasing/bullying/daring
(Possible solutions: refer to school 'anti-bullying policy'; be assertive, tell a parent/teacher/friend.) See also 'Zero tolerance!' on page 44.

■ homework
(Possible solutions: always ask straight away if you don't understand what you have to do; write down instructions; find a quiet place to work; don't leave it until the last minute; take your time!)

■ exams/tests
(Possible solutions: make sure you are clear about what you are going to be tested on; ask to go through past papers in class; practise exam techniques such as reading the question very carefully first, allowing enough time to answer each question, leaving anything you are stuck on until last and so on; allocate time for revision; keep calm.) See also 'Test survival skills' on page 60.

■ future employment
(Possible solutions: value school and qualifications; develop social skills such as teamwork, politeness, consideration for others, reliability and perseverance; take up hobbies and interests to develop different skills.)

OBJECTIVES
To enable children to:
■ develop self-insight
■ recognize when they are worried about something
■ cope with difficult emotions and fears
■ distinguish between real and imaginary worries
■ know who to approach for help with a worry.

CROSS-CURRICULAR LINKS
ENGLISH
Communicating effectively in speech; formulating, analysing and expressing ideas; discussing possibilities; drama.

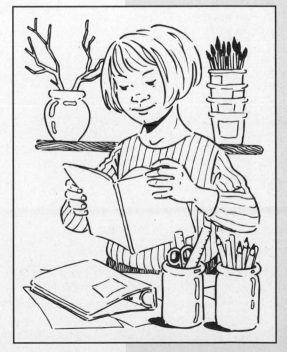

To end on a positive note, ask the groups to brainstorm some hopes for the future of their character – from ideas for careers to ambitions such as travelling to exotic countries and so on.

Ask the children to consider how they felt about today's activity. Did they feel relieved to talk about how to deal with worries? What have they learned about worries and how to tackle them? How can they apply this in everyday life? Emphasize that everyone has worries, but 'a worry shared is a worry halved' – there is always someone you can approach for help. It is not silly to have worries. If you don't tell anyone, they may not realize that you are worried about something.

NOW OR LATER

■ Ask small groups to devise some mini dramas to show children with worries successfully sorting them out.

■ The class could collaborate to produce a book about worries and their solutions which might be shared with parents or other classes, and kept available if children want to refer to it at any time.

■ If a particular worry has been frequently mentioned, set up a noticeboard display about it. For example, ex-pupil's comments about the local secondary schools could be put up, together with photographs.

MOOD MUSIC

OBJECTIVES

To enable children to:
■ express feelings and emotions in different ways
■ understand what triggers some emotions
■ recognize and name different feelings
■ manage feelings and emotions positively
■ recognize that people may respond differently to the same stimulus.

CROSS-CURRICULAR LINKS

ENGLISH

Formulating, clarifying and expressing ideas; describing experiences; developing vocabulary; extended writing; drama.

MUSIC

Responding to music; listening with concentration; recognizing how sounds are used in music to achieve particular effects; improvising musical patterns; using sounds to create musical effects; communicating musical ideas to others; responding to musical elements and changing the character or mood of a piece of music by means of dance or other forms of expression.

ART

Expressing ideas and feelings.

RESOURCES AND CLASSROOM ORGANIZATION

Select in advance some pieces of music on CD or cassette (some suggestions are given on the opposite page). You will also need: a CD or cassette player to play the music to the class; paper; art and writing materials.

Children listen to music as a class, then work individually and end with a class discussion.

WHAT TO DO

Explain to the class that they are going to be asked to listen really carefully to a piece of music, and then to make a 'portrait' of the music to express the mood it inspires in them.

Play a slow, calm, thoughtful piece of music (melancholy, wistful, poignant…) *or* a happy, triumphant piece (joyful, exciting, celebratory…) *or* an amusing piece (hilarious, comical, droll…) *or* a sinister piece (menacing, foreboding, eerie…).

After listening to the music several times, if necessary, ask the children to construct a picture (fairly quickly) from the colours, shapes or textures they feel are evoked by the music.

Ask each child to add words or phrases to their pictures to enhance the mood they want to express. Display the pictures. Did children have different ideas about the mood created, or are they all similar? You may want to repeat the exercise with a contrasting piece of music.

Now discuss with the class how the composers have created certain effects in the pieces of music. Talk about the pace and volume, which instruments are used and how they are played, for example bowing or plucking strings, and about the use of major and minor keys. The lyrics of appropriate songs can be analysed too, to discover evocative words and phrases.

Talk about *when* and *how* people use different pieces of music. *Why do they want to create a particular atmosphere such as at weddings, funerals or parties?* Move on to discuss how music can affect the mood we are in and indeed how it can have a powerful effect on our feelings.

End by asking the children what they have learned about music and feelings and how they could use this knowledge in everyday life, for example by playing lively music to energize themselves or by listening to a calming piece of music for relaxation.

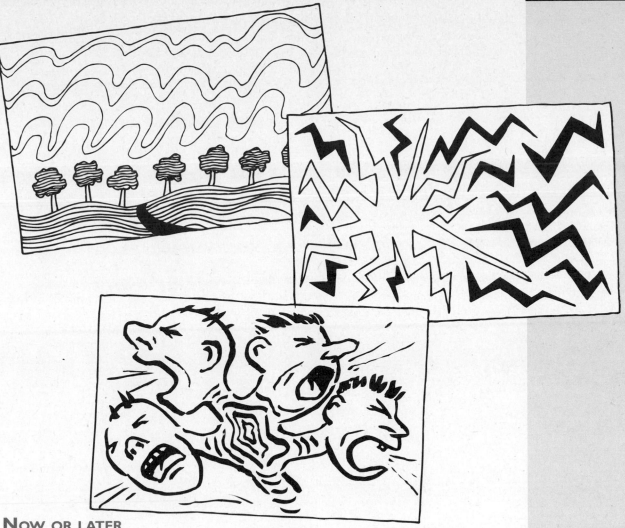

NOW OR LATER

■ Ask the children to write down the names of the composers and the pieces of music which they have heard and describe their feelings and what they were reminded of, using as wide a vocabulary as possible.

■ Children could compose their own mood music in pairs or small groups and perform it to the class, perhaps with accompanying dance or drama.

■ The children could create a mood painting for a chosen piece of music and design an appropriate CD cover for it.

■ A combination of the above work would make a good theme for an assembly or other presentation.

MUSIC SUGGESTIONS

Triumphant, happy, joyful
Dvořák: *Carnival* overture
Smetena: *Valtava*
Handel: *Water Music*
Robbie Williams: 'Millennium' from *I've Been Expecting You*

Relaxing, soothing and/or sad, thoughtful
JS Bach: 'Jesu, Joy Of Man's Desiring'
Pachelbel: *Canon and Gigue in D*

Beethoven: Sonata No 14 – Second movement *(Moonlight)*
Elgar: *Variations on an original theme (Enigma)* – No 9 'Nimrod'
Madonna: 'Frozen' from *Ray of Light*

Sinister, frightening, foreboding
Mussorgsky: *Night on the Bare Mountain*
Holst: 'Mars, the Bringer of

War' from *The Planets* suite
John Williams: theme music for the film *Jaws*

Amusing
Vivaldi: Concerto for Double Bassoon
Rimsky-Korsakov: *Flight of the Bumble Bee*
Haydn: Symphony No 94 *(Surprise)*
Leopold Mozart: *Toy Symphony*

Photocopiables

1

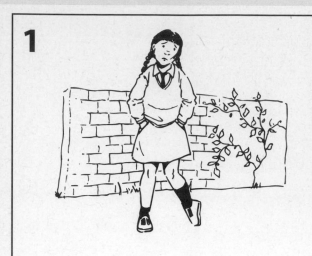

_____

2

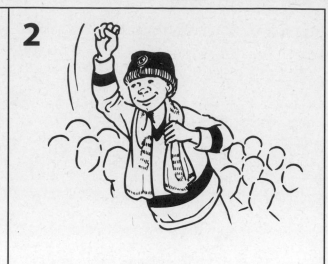

_____

3

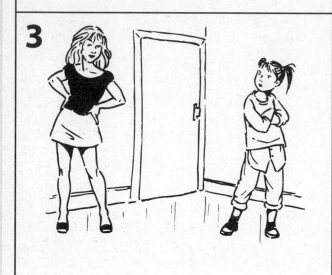

_____

4

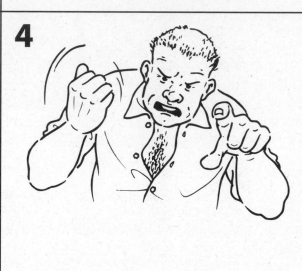

_____

5

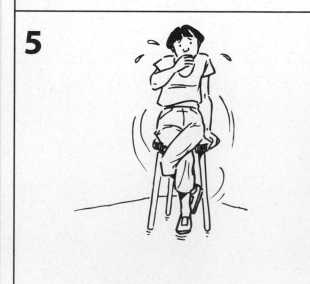

_____

6

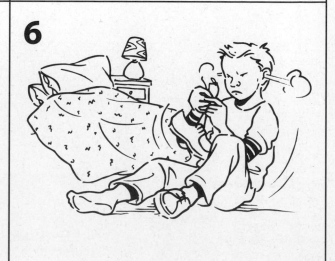

_____

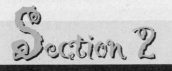 **Section 2**

DEVELOP A HEALTHY LIFESTYLE

The activities in this section focus on children:
- learning about factors which keep them healthy, and making healthy choices
- influencing the school as a health-promoting community
- acquiring personal hygiene skills
- taking pride in their own bodies
- appreciating the importance of safe food-handling
- understanding the work of health professionals.

BE NICE TO KNOW!

RESOURCES AND CLASSROOM ORGANIZATION

You will need: a copy of photocopiable page 20 for each child, enlarged if possible; board or flip chart; writing materials.

There is an initial class discussion followed by group work.

WHAT TO DO

Explain to the class that they are going to find out about something called 'personal hygiene'. Write this on the board. Ask: *What does 'hygiene' mean?* (Keeping everything really clean and 'hygienic', for example in kitchens, keeping surfaces and sinks clean so that microbes such as harmful bacteria are not passed from one thing to another.) *What would an 'unhygienic' kitchen look like?* (Scraps of food left out, grubby cloths, dirty surfaces and so on.) *So what do you think we mean by 'personal hygiene'?* (Keeping ourselves and our clothes clean and 'nice to know'.)

Explain that as we grow up, during puberty, our skin changes. Sweat glands produce more sweat of a different kind, which if left on skin or clothes is acted on by bacteria and begins to smell unpleasant. The oil glands (sebaceous glands) in the skin also become more active, so skin and hair may become more greasy and need washing more often. Because of all these changes it's useful to plan ahead and practise good hygiene routines in advance!

Give each child a copy of photocopiable page 20, check their understanding of 'plaque', then ask them to work in small groups to discuss each 'message', and suggest some answers.

OBJECTIVES

To enable children to develop the skills for:
- personal hygiene
- making healthy choices
- taking pride in their own bodies
- taking responsibility for themselves.

CROSS-CURRICULAR LINKS

ENGLISH
Listening with understanding; discussing possibilities; making simple, clear explanations of choices.

SCIENCE
Keeping healthy; understanding micro-organisms.

MATHS
Solving problems, including situations involving money.

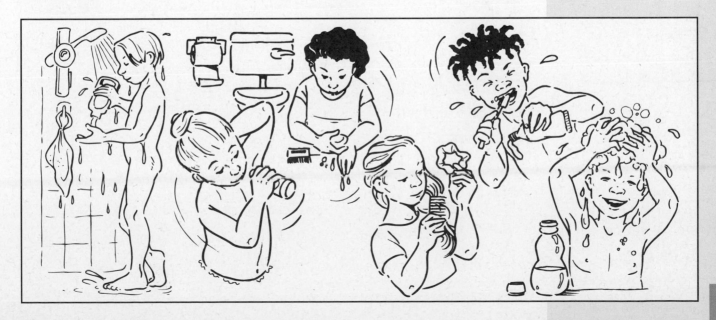

Answers to 'Be nice to know!' on photocopiable page 20

Skin. *We will:*
- frequently wash you all over using soap
- pay special attention to armpits and use an antiperspirant or deodorant if necessary
- cover cuts until they heal.

Hands. *We will always keep nails short and clean, and wash you:*
- after using the toilet
- before eating or preparing food
- after playing outside.

Mouth. *We will:*
- brush teeth twice a day to remove plaque
- use a fluoride toothpaste to strengthen teeth
- visit the dentist at least twice a year.

Hair. *We will:*
- brush and comb you
- shampoo you often (we will use an anti-dandruff shampoo if necessary)
- tie you back or get you cut if you get in our eyes.

Feet. *We promise to keep toenails short and clean, and*
- make sure our shoes and socks are big enough
- wash you and dry carefully between our toes
- wear clean socks/tights every day.

Openings between our legs. *We will take care of you by*
- wiping you properly after using the toilet (girls should wipe from front to back)
- washing you carefully and often
- wearing clean pants every day.

For the last 'message' you might like to comment that it's quite usual to feel a bit embarrassed when talking about parts of our bodies we don't normally mention in public! Say: *So let's have a good giggle and get the embarrassment out of the way. Now we can think sensibly about keeping **all** parts of our body clean.*

Be aware that one in ten girls start their periods while at primary school (some when only nine). They might appreciate an informal chat with the school nurse, or a volunteer mum, about menstrual hygiene and how to cope at school. All schools should check that they have made appropriate provision for pubertal girls. (See also solutions to worries in the activity 'Looking ahead – hopes and fears' on page 9.)

Ask each group to explain one of their solutions, for class discussion. Each child can add any extra ideas to the back of the photocopiable sheet.

NOW OR LATER

- You may like to raise discussion of 'special situations' which are commonly encountered in young children, such as dealing with threadworms (40 per cent of children under ten have them at some time), necessitating medication, extra hand-washing, keeping nails short and so on, and knowing how to cope with headlice, using a 'Sackers' comb to remove the eggs, and possibly a special shampoo as recommended by a health professional.
- Children could bring in items for a hygiene noticeboard, for example advertisements or packets, soap wrappers, empty shampoo bottles, and work out value for money and the cost of 'one wash'.
- The class could write an advice sheet for children their age, about how to keep all parts clean and 'nice to know'.

FOOD SAFETY

OBJECTIVES

To enable children to:
- understand under what conditions microbes multiply
- learn the skills for safe food-handling
- influence the school as a health-promoting community.

RESOURCES AND CLASSROOM ORGANIZATION

The 'Introduction to microbes' text (see page 15), written out on a large sheet of paper or as an overhead transparency; a copy of photocopiable page 21 for each child or pair; writing materials.

Following a class discussion, children work in pairs, then the whole class get back together to discuss answers.

WHAT TO DO

Introduce the topic by asking: *Has anyone heard of salmonella?* Explain that it is a bacterium (a microbe) which is one of the most common causes of food poisoning, so it is really important that everyone understands about microbes. Now read the following introduction with the class, checking understanding of the words in italic.

Introduction to microbes

Micro-organisms or *microbes* (bacteria, viruses and some fungi) are minute living things which are all around us, but so small that we can't see them. Some are helpful to us and are used to make cheeses, yoghurts and yeast breads. Others usefully *decompose* and rot away any *biodegradable* waste such as orange peel, grass cuttings or dead leaves. However, some micro-organisms (often called 'germs') on or in foods can be harmful if we eat them, because they make us ill.

Micro-organisms can *thrive* in the warm, and at about 20°C are able to multiply very quickly, and can double their number every 20 minutes! If we eat food containing too many harmful microbes we can become ill with food poisoning. To stop microbes multiplying we must keep food either really hot (above 63°C) or cold (0–5°C for a fridge, and –18°C for freezers).

Give each child a copy of photocopiable page 21 and ask them (working in pairs) to fill in the blanks in the sentences. The number alongside each word space shows where to fill it in on the word puzzle. (All the words go down only.)

Answers to food safety puzzle on photocopiable page 21

1. meat, 2. fridge, 3. cooked, 4. raw, 5. foods, 6. mouldy, 7. fresh, 8. burgers, 9. washed, 10. utensils, 11. flies, 12. stored, 13. middle, 14. poisoning. The hidden word is *micro-organisms*.

Continuing as a class, go over the answers and discuss what they have learned. Ask: *How can we apply this to our everyday lives?* For example, can they explain how they would safely store the ingredients for, and safely prepare, a cheese sandwich? What about food brought into school? Where might the best and worst storage places be, and why?

NOW OR LATER

■ Let the children visit the school kitchen and talk to staff about food safety (help them to prepare questions in advance – for example, what temperature are the fridges?).

■ Ask the children to find out more about particular topics, such as houseflies, by doing research in the library or by using a CD-ROM.

■ Produce mini-dramas in groups. For example, a family having a Sunday lunch of chicken become very ill afterwards; the doctor/environmental health officer explains that the chicken was not fully defrosted and cooked right through to the middle, so the microbes survived!

■ Invite the children to bring in labels from various foods, microwave dishes and so on, and note the instructions, such as 'Keep refrigerated', 'Store below 5°C', 'Make sure it is thoroughly cooked'.

■ Use thermometers to discover the temperature in the classroom, (a) by a draught, (b) in the middle of the room, (c) by a radiator, and (d) inside a fridge. Draw a large thermometer and mark key temperatures on it.

■ Ask each child to draw one microbe, as a dot, in the centre at one end of a large sheet of paper and work out how many microbes there would be after two hours, if the numbers doubled every 20 minutes. (The answer is 64.) *What implications does this have for food safety if we assume that there can be hundreds of microbes on some foods?* Display the class results, for example for 30 children, 30 microbes after two hours would become 1920!

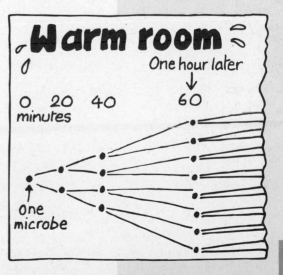

CROSS-CURRICULAR LINKS

ENGLISH
Giving reasons for opinions and actions; predicting outcomes and discussing possibilities; developing vocabulary; using reference books.

SCIENCE
Understanding micro-organisms and food safety; using thermometers.

MATHS
Problem-solving.

HEALTHY TUCK-SHOP PROJECT

OBJECTIVES

To enable children to:
- learn about factors which keep them healthy, and make healthy choices
- handle food safely
- enjoy healthy eating
- influence the school as a health-promoting community.

CROSS-CURRICULAR LINKS

ENGLISH

Formulating, clarifying and expressing ideas; sharing ideas; writing for varied purposes; extended writing.

MATHS

Solving problems, including situations involving money; collecting, recording and interpreting data, and presenting it in different forms.

SCIENCE

Learning about health and growth, teeth and eating, keeping healthy, micro-organisms, safe food-handling.

DESIGN & TECHNOLOGY

Using information sources to help in designing; generating ideas; considering users and purposes.

ICT

Using ICT equipment to carry out a variety of functions in a range of contexts; entering and storing information; retrieving, processing and displaying stored information.

GEOGRAPHY

Understanding about links with other places, for example supply of food.

RESOURCES AND CLASSROOM ORGANIZATION

You will need: a large sheet of paper; writing materials; adult supervision of stock handling if ideas are implemented.

Children work in groups, then as a class.

WHAT TO DO

Explain to the class that they are going to consider how to set up a healthy tuck-shop for the school. *Why is it important that if we have snacks between meals they are healthy ones?* (Answers may include: low sugar snacks are better for teeth; low fat is healthier for the heart; fresh fruit and vegetables are important for vitamins; low salt is healthier for blood pressure; high fibre is good for our digestive system.)

Divide the children into small groups and ask them to discuss and write down all the things they would have to think about in order to set up a tuck-shop. Give a couple of examples from the list below. To encourage the children, explain that groups will be awarded a point for each appropriate idea.

Checklist:
- Which foods and drinks will be sold? (Apples, bananas, mineral water?)
- Where will these be bought from, how often and by whom?
- How will they be stored safely and securely?
- Where will the tuck-shop be and when will it be open?
- How should perishable food like fruit and cherry tomatoes be handled? (Fruit and hands should be washed.)
- How will the goods be displayed?
- How will a rota be made for children serving in the tuck-shop, and for adult supervision?
- How should they advertise the shop?
- Who will design and produce advertisements/posters and so on, and a price list?
- Who decides whether to make a profit (for school funds?) and if so, how large should the 'mark up' be?
- How would accounts be kept and by whom?
- How would money be handled and stored? If it is to be in a bank account, who would open the account and run it?

After about 15 minutes, ask each group in turn for their suggestions and write each valid idea on a large sheet of paper. Give each group one point for every useful idea they thought of. Which group did best?

The class could now use the final list to *either* get adult help to plan and set up a tuck-shop *or* find out from those running one already how they have coped with all

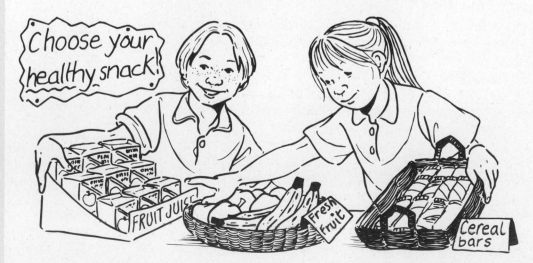

the considerations raised. Could any changes be made to what's on offer to provide a healthier choice?

Finally, the children can be asked what they have learned about working in groups, sharing ideas, getting information, obtaining healthy snacks and so on, and how they will be able to use this knowledge and these health skills in their everyday lives.

NOW OR LATER

■ As a design & technology project, children could design posters for the tuck-shop, as well as price lists and so on. They can then use a desktop publishing package to produce the posters and also use the computer for keeping money records.

■ Ask the children to write in detail about the benefits of the healthy foods and drinks on offer at the tuck-shop, and about safe food-handling.

■ Link buying, selling, counting money and giving change to a maths topic.

■ As part of a geography project, children could find out from where in the world the tuck-shop food originated, and show these places on a map.

■ Ask the children to write about their experiences – the planning, the setting up and the running of the shop – and include illustrations and computer printouts. This can be presented in book form or as a noticeboard display, with suggestions for future groups.

EVERY BODY IS DIFFERENT

RESOURCES AND CLASSROOM ORGANIZATION

In advance, ask the children to collect pictures of men and women from advertisements in magazines and newspapers. You will also need: a table on which to spread out the pictures; paper; writing materials.

Children work as a whole class.

WHAT TO DO

Display the collected pictures on the table. Discuss the similarities and differences between the people depicted. Explain: *We are going to be talking about different body types, but we will not mention people we know, as this can be hurtful.* Ask: *Do you think the range of body types you can see accurately resemble those you see in real life?* (Probably, no.) *Are there ways in which the bodies are different? Is there a range of height, shape and skin colour? Do they show old or small people? When people change into adults, do you think they have any control over what their final body shape will be?* (They have some control due to the amount of exercise they take and the type and quantity of food they eat, but a lot of features are inherited – height, shape and, to some degree, size.)

Ask the children: *How do the advertising images of men's and women's bodies compare with reality?* (Females are generally much taller and slimmer than 'average', and young and good looking. Men are often 'macho', with bulging muscles.) *Do you think that constantly seeing such images makes us all have an 'ideal' image of what a 'perfect' body is and what everyone should strive for in order to be successful?* Discuss what problems this might cause, and explain what is meant by 'stereotypes'. People become unhappy with the way they look; they try to change themselves, for example by dieting when they are not really overweight instead of just trying to be as healthy as they can. Explain that an obsession with being really thin, like models on the catwalk and in magazines, can lead to eating problems. Perhaps you could mention anorexia nervosa and bulimia, and that help is available for these conditions. Ask: *What can we learn from all this?* (That the media can put pressure on us.) *Should we try harder to accept everyone the way they are, regardless of size and shape?*

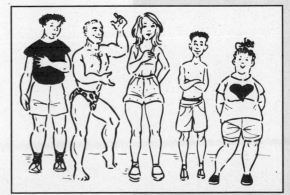

OBJECTIVES
To enable children to:
■ take pride in their own bodies
■ resist inappropriate pressures
■ respect differences between people
■ question media images and stereotypes.

CROSS-CURRICULAR LINKS
ENGLISH
Communicating effectively in speech and writing; formulating, clarifying and expressing ideas.

17

Finish by asking the children to write down what they have learned about advertisers' choice of body shapes and how this might be useful in the future.

NOW OR LATER

■ Prepare a noticeboard display using the pictures collected and ask the children to add comments on the differences between the fantasy of advertisements and reality.
■ For homework, ask the children to watch out for the selection of body types used in television advertisements to see if what they learned about magazine adverts applies to other media. Other aspects could be identified and discussed, for example are all fat people treated as figures of fun? Are very tall people referred to as 'lofty'?
■ Start a collection of photographs of successful people who do not conform to stereotypical images.

WHY EXERCISE?

OBJECTIVES

To enable children to:
■ learn about factors which keep them healthy, and make healthy choices
■ learn about the many benefits of exercise
■ have pride in their own bodies.

CROSS-CURRICULAR LINKS

ENGLISH

Making simple clear explanations of choices; giving reasons for opinions and actions; sharing ideas, insights and opinions.

SCIENCE

Developing understanding of how to keep healthy; knowing about the importance of exercise (for health).

PE

Learning how to be physically active and how to have a healthy lifestyle.

RESOURCES AND CLASSROOM ORGANIZATION

You will need: a copy of photocopiable page 22 for each child; writing materials.
Class discussion leads into individual work, with a final reflective session.

WHAT TO DO

Introduce the activity to the children by asking them: *Why should we exercise?* (Answers might include: to keep fit and stay healthy; make and keep our muscles strong and bodies supple; make and keep our heart and lungs strong and healthy; help us 'keep in shape'/stay a healthy weight; reduce tension and stress; feel good about ourselves.)

Now ask: *How often, according to health professionals, should we take exercise?* (Ideally for about 20 minutes, three times a week.) This should involve becoming slightly out of breath; if this happens, we know we have put in enough effort for the exercise to be effective.

Then ask: *What sort of exercise can we do?* (There should be a wide range of responses: team sports – football, netball, cricket, hockey and so on – running, jogging, brisk walking, cycling, swimming, athletics, gymnastics, aerobics, gym workouts.) *How can we choose the right exercise for us?* (Answers might include: an exercise that we can enjoy; do locally (that is, get to easily); do with friends; do on our own, if preferred; fit into our weekly routine; an exercise that involves competing/not competing, with others.)

Next, give out copies of photocopiable page 22 and ask the children to complete the questionnaire to help them 'commit to get fit'.

Conclude the activity by asking the children what they have learned and how important they feel this might be for their future health.

NOW OR LATER

■ Conduct a follow-up session in which children volunteer to tell the class how they have increased the amount of exercise they take.

■ Suggest that the children collect pictures of their favourite exercise/sport and sports personalities to produce a noticeboard display encouraging people to take more exercise.

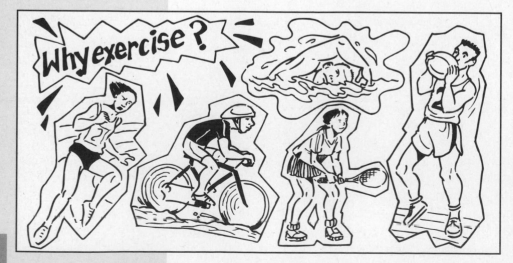

GET ORGANIZED!

RESOURCES AND CLASSROOM ORGANIZATION

You will need: a set of seven blank rectangular stickers for each child; A4 paper; rulers; writing and colouring materials

After an initial discussion, children work individually, then have a closing class discussion.

WHAT TO DO

Ask the children how they feel when they are late or when they have forgotten to do something. Ask them: *Why does it help to be organized?* (Because it saves everyone time and worry, and means we won't forget things as often.) *What sorts of things do we need to remember?* (When to hand in homework, bring in our swimming things, return a book, go to the dentist, and so on.)

Give each child a set of blank stickers and a sheet of A4 paper. Tell them that they are going to make themselves a weekly planner and put on 'reminders' to remind them of important days and dates – these will be their own ideas drawn on the blank stickers. Explain the following instructions to the children:

■ Measure the short side of your A4 sheet and divide it into eight sections. Rule lines across for the heading and days of the week.

■ Now rule four columns going down the page. Fill in your name and the headings 'Morning', 'Afternoon' and 'Evening', then the days of the week.

■ Plan the week ahead, deciding what you will need to remember and when. Make your own reminders by writing on the blank stickers, perhaps adding little designs and colouring them in. Fix each completed sticker to the appropriate section of the organizer.

Name	Morning	Afternoon	Evening
Monday			
Tuesday			
Wednesday			
Thursday			
Friday			
Saturday			
Sunday			

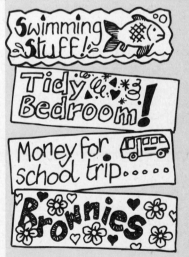

When everyone has finished, ask volunteers to tell the class about the reminders they have put on their planners. Suggest that they place the organizer in a prominent position at home and check it each evening so that they can get things ready for the next day. Summarize by asking the children what they have learned about what it means to be organized.

NOW OR LATER

■ Children could mount their organizers onto card, and share ideas about other ways of being organized – writing lists, using Post-it notes, using a calendar, having a regular time each week for getting particular tasks done.

■ Make a class planner including times of lessons, dates of school trips, concerts and other events, and display it in the classroom.

■ Groups could write and/or act out stories about 'Muddled Melissa' or 'Disorganized Darren', and their counterparts, 'Penny Planner' and 'Tidy Tim'!

OBJECTIVES

To enable children to:
■ learn about factors which make them healthy, and make healthy choices
■ understand the importance of being organized
■ develop skills to get organized.

CROSS-CURRICULAR LINKS

ENGLISH

Writing in response to a wide range of stimuli, including classroom activities.

MATHS

Using purposeful contexts for measuring.

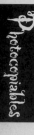

Be nice to know!

Messages from	Our replies
Our skin I protect you from knocks and germs. As you grow up, I will sweat more, especially under your arms. I warn you that some microbes act on the sweat and make it smell!	This calls for skinny dipping! We will… ■ ■ ■
Our hands Every day we touch many things for you, but pick up germs which could make you ill.	We will always keep nails short and clean, and wash you… ■ ■ ■
Our mouth I am busy growing your new permanent teeth. I'm worried about the microbes in your plaque that can damage teeth and gums and cause bad breath!	Don't worry mouth! Smile! We will… ■ ■ ■
Our hair As you grow up, I will help you look great, but I could get rather oily for a while!	Hair we go! We will… ■ ■ ■
Our feet We grow fast and need more space. We sweat a lot and hate smelly socks!	Don't fret feet! We promise to keep toenails short and clean, and… ■ ■ ■
Our openings between our legs You need us to get rid of wastes. As you grow up, this area will sweat more. To stay healthy we must be clean and dry.	Fear not! We will take care of you by… ■ ■ ■

Food safety puzzle

Foods such as **m**_____ (**1**), cheese and yoghurts should be kept cold in a

f_____ (**2**) so that microbes can multiply only slowly and the food stays

f_____ (**7**). Food should be covered so that **f**_____ (**11**)

cannot land on it and infect it with microbes from their feet. Meat such as chicken and

b_____ (**8**) should be thoroughly **c**_____ (**3**) and checked

before eating to make sure it is not still raw in the **m**_____ (**13**).

All **u**_____ (**10**) (knives, forks, spoons) that have touched food should be

w_____ (**9**) in hot water with detergent to kill the micro-organisms.

R_____ (**4**) foods and cooked **f**_____ (**5**) should always be

s_____ (**12**) (kept) separately, so microbes from the raw food do not get

onto the cooked food. Drier foods such as bread should be stored in a cool, dry place

so they don't go **m**_____ (**6**) (furry looking spots appear!). If we follow all

these guidelines, we have much less chance of becoming ill because of the micro-

organisms in our food which can cause food **p**_____ (**14**).

■ Fill in the missing words, then write them in the puzzle. They all read downwards.

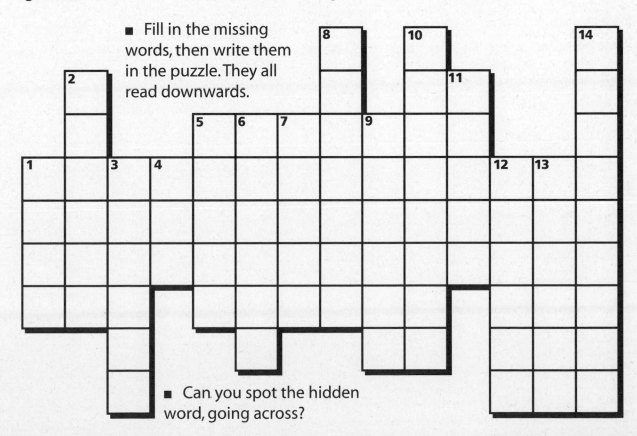

■ Can you spot the hidden word, going across?

Photocopiables

I commit to get fit!

1. I would like to take regular exercise to: *(Tick those that apply to you.)*

(a) keep fit and healthy ☐

(b) keep my muscles, heart and lungs strong and healthy ☐

(c) keep 'in shape' and the right weight for me ☐

(d) feel great! ☐

2. I am going to try and exercise on the following days of the week:

_____

_____

_____

3. I would like to choose an exercise that is: *(Tick those that apply.)*

(a) enjoyable ☐

(b) local ☐

(c) sociable – with friends ☐

(d) competitive ☐

(e) not competitive ☐

(f) *(Fill in your description.)*

_____

_____

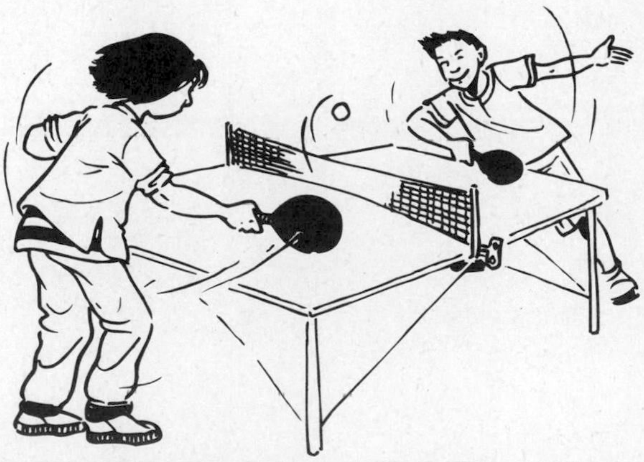

4. The following exercises appeal to me:

football ☐

netball ☐

hockey ☐

cricket ☐

cycling ☐

swimming ☐

badminton ☐

short tennis ☐

tennis ☐

table tennis ☐

horse-riding ☐

jogging ☐

aerobics ☐

exercise machines ☐

circuit training ☐

squash ☐

brisk walking ☐

other(s) _____

_____

5. I commit to get fit! So I will arrange to do the following:

_____

_____

_____

_____

_____

_____

Signed _____

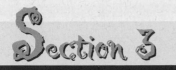

Section 3

LEARN TO KEEP THEMSELVES AND OTHERS SAFE

The activities in this section focus on children:
- being aware of hazards to health and safety
- assessing risks
- learning safety skills
- knowing where to get help
- resisting pressure.

HELPFUL OR HAZARDOUS?

RESOURCES AND CLASSROOM ORGANIZATION

Prepare in advance a collection of empty packets and cartons from 'over the counter' non-prescription medicines (for example, cough medicines, pain relievers), enough for children to work in pairs with one product. You will also need: a copy of photocopiable page 27 for each child; writing materials.

Children work in pairs, with a class discussion before and after the activity.

WHAT TO DO

Explain that the children are going to work in pairs on a task which will help them find out about how to work with their families to use medicines safely. Warn the class that no child should take any medicines or drugs without adult supervision, unless they have been specially trained (for example, children with asthma will have been shown how to use an inhaler).

Give each child a copy of photocopiable page 27, and each pair one *empty* medicine packet. Ask them to read and discuss the instructions on the packet which grown-ups have to read, and to fill in their photocopiable sheet as best they can, ticking the boxes and writing on the answer lines.

Follow this with a class discussion of their findings. Stress that reading instructions is important, dosage *does* matter (it is carefully worked out for different sizes and ages, and 'more' is *not* better, as medicines can have side-effects). All 'over the counter' medicines and drugs from pharmacists have been carefully tested, so warnings should be heeded and advice sought if in doubt.

Explain that not all drugs are medicines. Illegal drugs may not be pure, have no instructions about dosage, side-effects or hazards. Proper medicines can help us *if* we use them correctly, take them only when they are really needed and only with adult help and according to instructions.

OBJECTIVES
To enable children to:
- learn about hazards to health and safety
- assess risks
- develop safety skills
- learn about appropriate use of medicines.

CROSS-CURRICULAR LINKS
ENGLISH
Reading different sources of information; writing in response to a variety of stimuli.

SCIENCE
Learning about keeping healthy; developing knowledge of drugs and medicines.

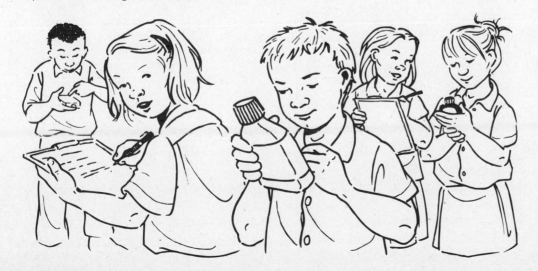

NOW OR LATER

■ The children could formulate a 'medicine code' for using medicines correctly, and write these on drawings of large medicine bottles for display.

■ Can the children find out more about how to store medicines safely? Ask: *What are 'child resistant' caps? What should you do if a child has swallowed medicines or tablets which were not for them?*

■ Link the activity to other areas in which children would need to think about safety. Ask the children to make a list of topics such as 'Road safety', 'Water safety', 'Safety around the school' and find out more about them.

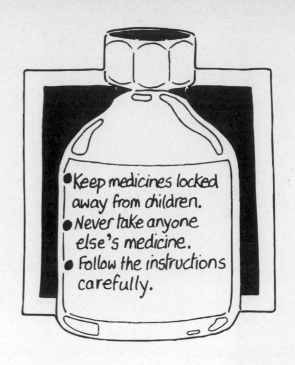

- Keep medicines locked away from children.
- Never take anyone else's medicine.
- Follow the instructions carefully.

BEING ASSERTIVE

OBJECTIVES

To enable children to:
■ learn about hazards to health and safety
■ develop skills for resisting pressure
■ know where to get help.

CROSS-CURRICULAR LINKS

ENGLISH

Exploring, developing and explaining ideas; sharing ideas, insights and opinions; reporting and describing events and observations; evaluating their own and others' ideas in responding to drama.

RESOURCES AND CLASSROOM ORGANIZATION

Prepare a set of situation cards for each group by making copies of photocopiable page 28 onto card and cutting out the cards. You will also need: board or flip chart; writing materials.

Children work as a class, then in groups of four, with a final class discussion.

WHAT TO DO

Explain to the children that they are going to learn about how people sometimes try and make us do things we don't want to and how we can use 'assertive' behaviour to stop them. Ask: *What does 'assertive' mean?* (Saying what you think and standing up for yourself firmly but politely, respecting the other person, but also knowing you have equal rights yourself.) So 'being assertive' does *not* mean 'being aggressive'!

Ask one of the children to come out to the front so that you can demonstrate the range of responses to someone pressurizing you to do something. Pretend to be rubbing out some writing on a sheet of paper. Ask the child to say, 'I want to borrow your rubber. Give it to me now.' Then respond in three different ways, illustrating and explaining:

■ *A passive response* which indicates that although you are using your rubber, you feel the other person has a greater right to it. Say, reluctantly, looking down, 'Alright, take it.' Explain how you feel like a victim.

■ *An aggressive response.* Say fiercely, fists up, (gently) pushing the child away, 'Absolutely no way! You never let me borrow yours!' This may start an argument and a fight!

■ *An assertive response.* Looking the child in the eyes, say firmly, 'You may borrow it in a minute when I've finished with it, if you promise to give it back straight away.' This asserts your rights, but acknowledges that the other person has needs too.

Make sure that everyone understands the difference in these responses and write the three types on the board.

Now explain that they are going to work in groups of four to consider how they might respond to a given 'situation'. Give a set of situation cards to each group and ask the children to select *one* situation, discuss it and decide what might be a passive, aggressive and an assertive response. Two children in the group should then take it in turns to role-play the situation in the three ways as demonstrated earlier, while the other two watch and comment. Suggest that assertive behaviour can include simply saying that you 'need more time to decide' or you 'need to ask someone else' or you 'need to know more about it'. Also, you can offer an alternative – for example, for alcohol: 'But I'd love some orange juice.' Write these strategies on the board for reference. Effective role-plays can be repeated for the whole class to see.

Summarize by asking the children to reflect on this session, and to consider how they could use these skills in real life in the future.

NOW OR LATER

■ Ask the children to think of their own 'situations' to discuss and role-play.
■ Role-plays could be developed into mini-dramas with costumes, props and so on for an assembly or open day.

GETTING WELL AGAIN

RESOURCES AND CLASSROOM ORGANIZATION

Check in advance the current regime for vaccinations in your area. You will need: flip chart or board; a copy of photocopiable page 29 for each pair or small group; dictionaries, writing materials.

A substantial class discussion is followed by small group work and a final class reflection.

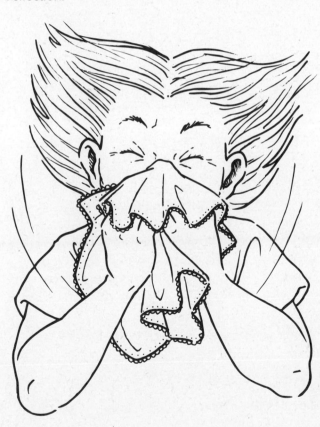

WHAT TO DO

Start the session by asking: *What travels at more than 100 mph and can reach up to 10 metres (30 feet) into the air?* (A sneeze!)

During the following dialogue, write all the underlined words on the board, with a short explanation next to each one (children can also look up definitions in a dictionary).

Ask: *Why is it a good idea to avoid being sneezed on?* (Because sneezes are made up of millions of tiny <u>droplets</u> which may contain <u>viruses</u>. If we breathe these in they may give us a cold or even flu (influenza). Viruses are just one of the <u>micro-organisms</u> (<u>microbes</u> or <u>germs</u>) which can cause <u>diseases</u> and make us ill.)

What other diseases can we catch? (Examples include chicken pox, warts, verrucas (all viruses) and diarrhoea and/or sickness, which can be from <u>bacteria</u>.)

Ask: *So what can we do about this?* (We can avoid being sneezed on, or sneezing on others; keep food safely, wash our hands carefully and often, and sometimes, if we have caught an illness, take medicines.)

Explain that if we have an illness caused by bacteria, the doctor might prescribe an <u>antibiotic</u> which will kill the bacteria and make us feel better, usually within a few days. Unfortunately, at the moment there are no antibiotics and very few other medicines that can kill viruses, so all we can do is to let our bodies fight them, and take

OBJECTIVES

To enable children to:
■ understand more about common illnesses
■ learn how to help themselves get better.

CROSS-CURRICULAR LINKS

ENGLISH
Sharing ideas, insights; exploring, developing and explaining ideas; dictionary work.

SCIENCE
Developing knowledge of micro-organisms, diseases and illnesses.

medicines to relieve the <u>symptoms</u>. Ask: *What do we feel like when we have a cold?* (Hot, tired, sore throat, headache, sneezy, runny nose/blocked nose, cough.) All these are symptoms and adults can help us by providing the right doses of pain relief (for example, paracetamol), throat sweets, vapour rub and so on. Our body's '<u>germ busting</u>' (immune) system usually takes about a week to ten days to fight off a cold virus, and we may need to keep warm and sometimes go to bed.

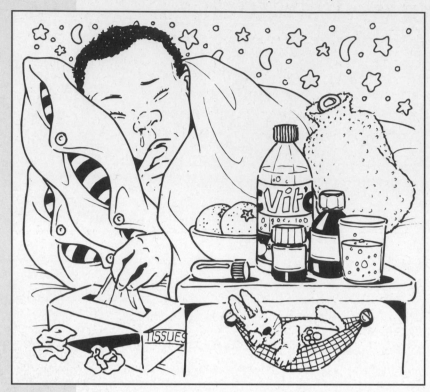

Now ask: Can *you think of any special ways doctors can help us not to get some diseases?* Explain that our National Health Service offers everyone the chance of being <u>vaccinated</u> against some of the diseases caused by bacteria (diphtheria, whooping cough [pertussis] and tetanus) and viruses (measles, rubella, mumps, polio and influenza). Doctors or nurses inject a special <u>vaccine</u> which is a 'pretend version' of the real disease. Our 'germ busting' system acts as though it were the real thing and makes a lot of <u>antibodies</u> to fight it. Then when we meet the real disease these antibodies are all ready, so we don't become ill.

Explain that there are certain 'conditions' which are *not* illnesses and *cannot* be caught from people who have them, for example asthma, eczema, hayfever, diabetes, epilepsy. These people need our support and friendship in helping them cope, and they are often experts in knowing what to do to help themselves and others.

Give out copies of photocopiable page 29 and ask the children to work in small groups. For each question they should choose the correct answer, and write the letter for it beside the question. Explain that each answer is used only once. More able children could be given the sheet with the answers blanked out, and paper on which to write the answers plus reference materials if appropriate.

Finally, ask the class to reflect on what they have learned. Reassure them that there are many things we can do to avoid getting ill. If we do get ill there are things we, and others, can do to help us get better as quickly as possible.

Answers to 'Getting well again' on photocopiable page 29			
1.	g	5.	a
2.	b, h	6.	c
3.	i	7.	f
4.	d	8.	e

NOW OR LATER

■ Arrange for the school nurse to explain more about vaccinations, how to cope with colds, or answer any other questions the children have prepared.

■ Ask the children to write stories and poems about 'A day in the life of a virus' or 'Feeling ill and getting better' or 'Billy the bacterium'.

■ In science, children could find out the range of 'normal' body temperatures and how high it may go during an illness.

■ Using books or CD-ROMs, children could research the work of Pasteur and Jenner, and find out about the beginning of the 'germ' theory of disease.

Taking care with medicines

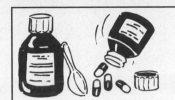

REMEMBER!
Medicines are not playthings.
Always ask an adult to help you.
Never take anyone else's medicine.

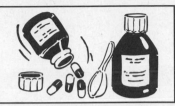

■ Read the instructions on the packet and answer as many questions as you can.

1. What is the *name* of the medicine? _____

2. What is it *used* for? _____

3. *How* should it be used?

   ☐ Swallowed   ☐ Inhaled   ☐ Rubbed in   Other _____

4. How much should be taken?

   None if aged _____ or under.

   Children 0–5 years _____

   Children 5–12 years _____

   Children 12 years and over _____

   Did you know that over half the cases of poisoning in children are because they have swallowed someone else's medicine?

5. *How often* should it be taken?

   _____ times a day   ☐ When needed   Every _____ hours

6. *When* should it be taken?

   ☐ Before meals   ☐ With food   ☐ After meals   ☐ Before bedtime   ☐ Other

7. Are there any *special instructions* to follow? _____

8. Are there any *warnings* about taking it, or about *side effects*? _____

9. Does it suggest you should see a *doctor* or *pharmacist* for further advice? _____

10. Do you think the *instructions* are *clear* and *easy* for everyone to understand?

Explain why/why not. _____

11. How should medicines be *stored* so that small children cannot get them? _____

_____

■ On a separate sheet, explain what you think *everyone* should know about taking medicines and storing them correctly.

Being assertive

A friend dares you to walk across a wobbly plank over a gushing stream.

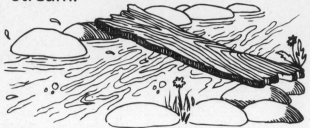

An older pupil at school tries to make you steal a packet of sweets from the local shop.

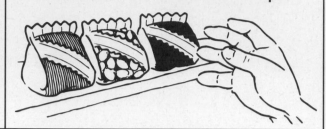

At a friend's house, when their parents are out, the friend offers you some alcohol to drink.

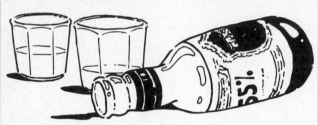

Your friend's older brother offers you a cigarette.

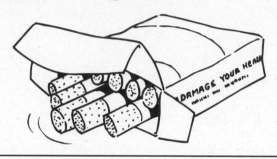

Your parents think you are at the cinema, but your friend wants to go for a take-away instead.

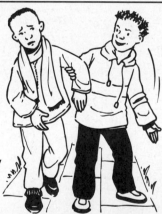

A bully in the playground tries to take your dinner money off you.

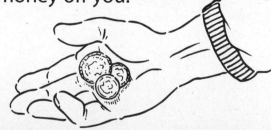

A friend wants you to try glue-sniffing with them.

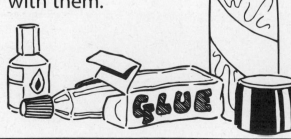

Your friend wants to kiss you but you don't want to kiss them.

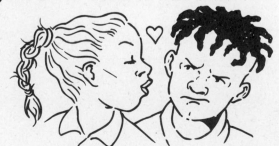

Ready to go! IDEAS FOR PSHE

Name   Date

Getting well again

1. Two illnesses caused by viruses are: ☐

2. Two things we can all do to prevent diseases spreading are: ☐ and ☐

3. How many sorts of cold virus are there? ☐

4. Three diseases we can be vaccinated against are: ☐

5. The name given to a medicine which kills bacteria is an: ☐

6. Three things we can do to help ourselves if we have a bad cold are: ☐

7. What can we do to cheer up someone who is ill? ☐

8. Three things we can do to keep our 'germ busting' system in good order are: ☐

Sort out the mixed-up microbes to find the right answers. Write the correct letter in each box.

a. antibiotic.

b. wash our hands often.

c. have lots of rest, plenty of drinks and keep warm and dry.

d. measles, mumps and rubella.

e. eat more fruit and vegetables, have plenty of exercise, get enough sleep.

f. Send a get well card.

g. polio and influenza.

h. only sneeze into 'a tissue'!

i. There are 200 types of cold virus.

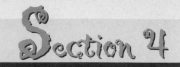

The activities in this section focus on children:
- reflecting on current relationships, friends and families
- considering future relationships and parenthood
- meeting, and developing relationships with, a variety of people
- working co-operatively and reflecting on their contribution to a group
- voicing different opinions sensitively; being courteous
- considering the needs of others and how their actions can have consequences for others.

TOGETHER – EVERYONE ACHIEVES MORE!

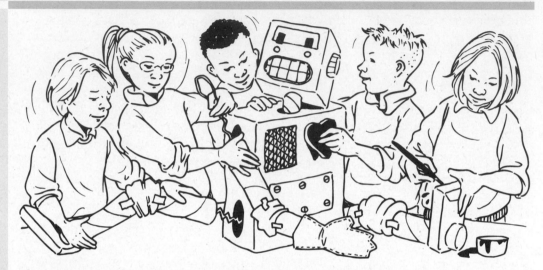

OBJECTIVES

To enable children to:
- learn how to co-operate with others
- reflect on their contribution to group working
- voice different opinions sensitively; be courteous
- consider the needs of others.

CROSS-CURRICULAR LINKS

ENGLISH

Taking turns in speaking; communicating effectively in speech and writing; qualifying or justifying what they think after listening to other opinions; dealing politely with opposing points of view; extended writing.

RESOURCES AND CLASSROOM ORGANIZATION

Prepare in advance materials for an activity which the children can do in groups and which involves several different tasks. For example, they could colour in, cut out and glue together a simple model printed on card or constructed from empty packets, boxes and so on.

Children work in groups, followed by a final class analysis of the process.

WHAT TO DO

Explain that the children are going to be divided into groups to complete an activity. They will be awarded points for how well they do. There will be a time-limit of about 30 minutes and you will be looking to see whose finished item is the best and who works well together as a team. Each group will have to decide whether they need a leader, and if so, choose one. They then need to decide who is to carry out each task.

Divide the class into groups of four or five. Give out the materials, explain the activity and say: *Your time starts now!* When the time is up, ask everyone to stop and listen. Go round the groups and award marks out of ten for how well the group co-operated, completed the task and tidied up.

Now ask the class about how well each group worked together. Did they easily decide on a leader? Did everyone agree, or was it a 'majority decision'? How did they decide who was to do each task, for example did people volunteer or did the leader tell them what to do? Did everyone do their fair share of the work? If not, why not? (They may not have been allocated much to do.) What other things need to be considered when working well as a group, for example who is good at which task? How did they as individuals contribute to the group – were they co-operative and helpful? Did everything go well? What were the problems (if any) and how did the group sort them out? What could have been done better? What would have happened if someone had refused to co-operate?

What three things have the children learned about how to work well in a group? How might this be useful in the future? (For school work, in a job/career.)

NOW OR LATER

■ Children could write up their experience of working in a group, answering the questions given above.

■ When asked to work as part of a group in another context, for example as a team for games in a PE lesson, children could be reminded about the benefits of co-operation as a group.

FRIENDSHIP UPS AND DOWNS

RESOURCES AND CLASSROOM ORGANIZATION

You will need: a copy of photocopiable page 35 and a notebook for each group; a large sheet of paper for class use; writing materials.

Children work initially in groups, and finish with a class discussion and brainstorm.

WHAT TO DO

Explain to the children that today they are going to talk about ups and downs in friendships and how we can cope with them. Ask them: *Do friendships always go smoothly?* (No!) *What sorts of things might happen to upset a friendship?* Keep it impersonal here: someone's friend might make a new friend, or they might have an argument, and so on. *Does this always mean the end of a friendship?* (No, hopefully – if someone acts thoughtfully they can keep their friend.)

Divide the class into groups, and give each group a copy of the four story starters on photocopiable page 35. Ask each group to discuss each story and suggest what could be done to resolve the situations. Children should consider how each of the characters in the stories might be feeling, and one person in the group should take notes about everything that has been proposed. Then as a class, consider each story in turn and ask the groups about their ideas.

What have the children learned about friendships? Brainstorm words and phrases and write them on a large sheet of paper. For example, 'Friendships mean: give and take, compromise, patience, listening, understanding, sensitivity to feelings, respect'. Relationships with different friends are different! How can they make use of this knowledge in future?

OBJECTIVES

To enable children to:
■ consider the needs of others and how their actions can have consequences for others
■ understand more about friendships and how they work
■ gain the skills for being a good friend
■ work co-operatively in a group.

CROSS-CURRICULAR LINKS

ENGLISH
Sharing ideas, insights and opinions; reading for information; writing in response to a classroom activity; extended writing.

ICT
Using a computer to print out information.

Notes on the story starters on photocopiable page 35

Sam and Peter
Sam could explain to Peter and Laurence how he is feeling. Peter and Laurence could make an effort to include Sam more. Sam could find some other friends to spend some of his time with – perhaps it is helpful to have more than one special friend.

Lola and Helen
Lola could ask Helen why she is upset. Lola could try not to boast about her presents, and talk to Helen about how they could play with them together. Helen could try and cheer up and join in with Lola's celebrations.

Daniel and Sunhil
Sunhil could think about how Daniel is feeling and not gloat over winning. They could agree to play something else. Disagreeing doesn't mean you have to stop being friends. Daniel could try and be a good loser!

Laura and Debbie
Laura and Debbie can become pen-pals and phone or e-mail each other. They might still be able to meet if their parents can make the arrangements. Things rarely stay the same for ever, we all have to learn to make new friends, but we can keep in touch with old ones.

NOW OR LATER

■ Individuals or groups could write down happy endings to the stories using the ideas that the class discussed.

■ Ask the children to write a short essay about 'Friendships: dos and don'ts', based on what they have found out. They could list the skills they think are needed to be a good friend – loyalty, honesty and so on.

■ Children could word-process the start of other short stories about friendship problems, to hand out to other groups for discussion.

■ More words, phrases and illustrations could be added to the 'brainstorm' sheet.

ASKING FOR HELP

OBJECTIVES

To enable children to:

■ reflect on current relationships, friends and families

■ find out who is available to ask for help with different problems

■ develop skills for persisting in getting help.

CROSS-CURRICULAR LINKS

ENGLISH

Exploring, developing and explaining ideas; communicating effectively in speech; drama – role-playing.

RESOURCES AND CLASSROOM ORGANIZATION

In advance, look up contact numbers for the local police, Childline and any other organizations to whom children could turn for help. You will also need: a sheet of paper for each child; a large sheet of paper for helpline numbers; board or flip chart; writing materials.

An initial class discussion leads on to small group work, followed by a final class reflection.

WHAT TO DO

Start by talking to the children about needing help. Everyone needs help from others from time to time. We need to know who are suitable people to ask, and how to ask them. What ideas do the children have about what help they might need? (Help with homework, with bullying, with illness, in an emergency, with a worry and so on.) List these on the board.

Who are the first people that the children could approach? They might suggest friends, family, relatives, teachers. Ask them to write their own checklist ('My personal help checklist') on a sheet of paper.

Who can offer more specialist help? Encourage the children to discuss situations for which it would be appropriate to contact the local police, Childline, a surgery, a clinic and so on, and add these numbers to their checklists. (These may not be the same for all children.) Remind them about the procedure for emergencies: dialling 999… and the importance of only calling in a genuine emergency.

Now suggest that sometimes the person we really want to talk to is not available. *Why might this be?* (They are away, out or busy, for example.) We need to learn to persist in asking for help – we should try someone else, go back later or wait patiently until they are able to speak to you. Divide the class into small groups to make up their own mini-dramas of a child seeking help from someone who isn't available. For example:

■ A child is asking a parent for help with homework,

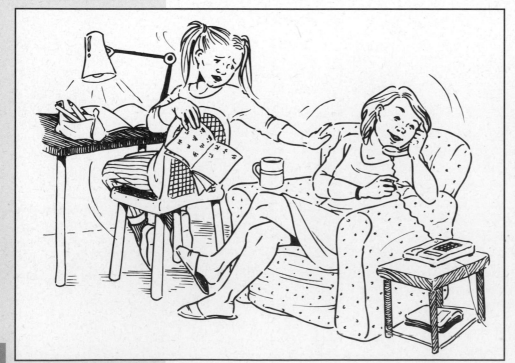

but Mum (parent, carer) is on the phone for a long time and can't give the child the attention he or she needs.

■ A child is trying to contact a teacher to explain he or she has not got the correct kit for the school match the next day, but the teacher is away on a day course.

Allow the children about ten minutes to work on their dramas. Explain that they should plan what the child will do next, such as wait for the adult and repeat the request or find another adult to help. Then let each group show their drama to the class for discussion. The class should note how many different ways of getting help have been suggested.

Conclude by asking the children what they have learned about asking for help. What techniques could they use in the future to persist until they get the help they need? (These may include talking to someone else instead, leaving an 'urgent' note on paper or perhaps sending an e-mail.)

NOW OR LATER

■ Children could also role-play getting help in an emergency, practising the correct procedure when dialling 999.

■ For homework, ask the children to research other useful telephone numbers, for example the number of an emergency plumber, a car breakdown service, a glazier.

EVERY PICTURE TELLS A STORY

RESOURCES AND CLASSROOM ORGANIZATION

Write the five 'situations' given below on an overhead transparency or flip-chart sheet. You will also need: a copy of photocopiable page 36 and a notebook or paper for each child; writing materials.

After a class introduction, children work in groups, before ending with a class discussion.

WHAT TO DO

Explain to the children that they are going to think about family or group situations in which each individual may be feeling something different. If we can imagine what someone else might be feeling it will help us to understand them better.

Give out copies of photocopiable page 36 and ask the children to look carefully at the picture and work out what they think has happened. Talk about possible answers to the questions and what might go in the speech bubbles. Divide the children into five groups and let them fill in their sheets together.

Now ask the children to consider what the same characters might be feeling in the following new situations and make notes about each, working in their groups:

■ The children come back from the disco one hour later than they promised to be home.

■ The children are moaning and complaining about having to visit their parents'/ carers' friends.

■ The children are asking for an increase in pocket money.

■ A parent is telling the children that it's time to go to bed, but they want to stay up to watch a television programme.

■ A parent is refusing to let the girl (or boy) have her (or his) ears pierced.

Ask each group to present their opinions on *one* of the situations. During the discussion, ask the class to decide what were the responsibilities of (1) the parent/ carer, and (2) the children, in each case. Can the children imagine what it must feel like to be a parent/carer themselves?

Conclude by encouraging the children to reflect on what they have discussed and ask: *What have you learned about the benefits of considering other people's feelings? What are the responsibilities of family members to each other? How might this knowledge be useful in the future?*

OBJECTIVES

To enable children to:
■ reflect on current relationships, friends and families
■ consider future relationships and parenthood
■ consider the needs of others and how their actions can have consequences for others
■ learn to respect others' feelings and needs.

CROSS-CURRICULAR LINKS

ENGLISH

Listening, understanding and responding appropriately to others; predicting outcomes and discussing possibilities; giving reasons for opinions.

NOW OR LATER

■ Children could draw their own pictures with speech bubbles or comic-strip style pictures to illustrate the scenarios they have discussed, or other situations they think of themselves.

■ Ask the children to list some points under the heading 'The responsibilities of parenthood' or 'The responsibilities of looking after other people'.

GREEN HATS, YELLOW HATS

OBJECTIVES

To enable children to:
■ consider the needs of others and how their actions can have consequences for others
■ reflect on current relationships
■ consider future relationships.

CROSS-CURRICULAR LINKS

ENGLISH

Exploring, developing and explaining ideas; sharing ideas, insights and opinions; writing in response to a range of stimuli, including classroom activities.

RESOURCES AND CLASSROOM ORGANIZATION

Prepare in advance some green and yellow paper hats, enough for half the class to wear one colour and the other half the other colour. You will also need: large sheets of 'graffiti' paper pinned up for 'feelings', headed 'When I wore a green hat I felt…', and 'When I wore a yellow hat I felt…'; a simple task for the children to do, such as cutting out all the different types of lettering that they can find from magazines, and sticking them onto a sheet.

Children work in two groups followed by a class discussion.

WHAT TO DO

Explain that the class will be divided into two groups, each wearing different coloured hats. They will be carrying out a task – tell them what this is. (They will start out wearing one colour hat, then change over halfway through.) Inform them that you, as the teacher, will have a particular role to play, but don't tell them what this is. Ask them to think about how they feel when they are wearing the green hats, and then the yellow hats (or vice versa).

Divide the class into two groups, give them their task and their coloured hats, and let them start work.

While they are working, go round everyone wearing a yellow hat and praise them, giving them lots of help. Ignore and 'dismiss' children wearing green hats. After 15 minutes or so, stop everyone and ask them to *think* how they are feeling, but not to comment on this or on your behaviour.

Swap over hats and repeat, so that for the next 15 minutes the previously 'ignored' children get all your attention.

Next, ask the children to think about the difference between the two groups and to record their feelings on the graffiti sheets. Lead the class discussion on their comments. How did they feel when wearing a yellow hat? (Reactions might include: important, successful, proud, happy, confident.) How did they feel when wearing the green hats? (Unimportant, a failure, hurt, sad, frustrated, angry, bewildered.)

What have the children learned from this? That everyone needs recognition and encouragement to feel good about themselves. Now ask them about the wider society and discuss who might be treated as if they were wearing yellow hats. (Beautiful people, rich people?) And who might be treated as if they were wearing green hats? (Ethnic minorities, people with disabilities, low-paid workers such as cleaners?)

Conclude by asking how the children might use their new understanding in the future – perhaps by showing appreciation for someone whom they have ignored in the past?

NOW OR LATER

■ Children could write about their experience in a green hat and yellow hat, and how they think this relates to a wider society.
■ Invite the children to make up their own role-play dramas to show people interacting positively with each other, for example a child appreciating a cooked meal; a child thanking the postman/woman who has just given him or her a letter; children acknowledging the crossing patrol who has helped them to cross the road.

Photocopiables

Friendship ups and downs

Sam and Peter

Sam and Peter have been best friends for years, since they started school together. Last week a new boy called Laurence joined their class, and Peter seems very friendly with him. Sam and Peter used to always play together, but now Peter sometimes plays with Laurence and forgets about Sam. Sam is starting to feel jealous and upset…

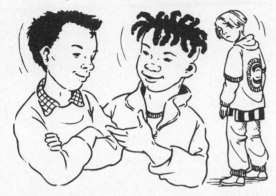

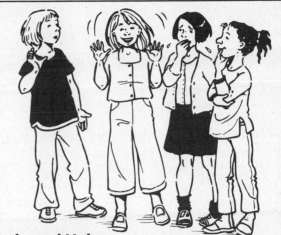

Lola and Helen

Lola and Helen sit next to each other and are always giggling happily together. Today is Lola's birthday and she is excited and telling everyone about the big expensive presents she has been given. Helen becomes quiet and a bit tearful as she remembers her own birthday…

Daniel and Sunhil

Daniel and Sunhil are playing football with their gang in the playground. Sunhil's side is winning and he scores a goal and jumps up, punching the air in triumph. Daniel feels miserable because he's losing. It's his football and he picks it up and walks away saying, "I've had enough. Let's play something else." Sunhil disagrees…

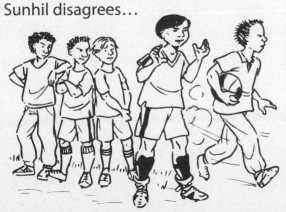

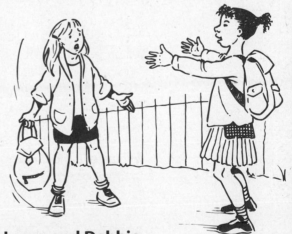

Laura and Debbie

Laura and Debbie who live across the street from each other have been best friends for many years. One day, Debbie comes into school with some exciting but disturbing news for Laura – her family are moving because her dad has a new job across the other side of the country…

Ready to go! IDEAS FOR PSHE

Every picture tells a story!

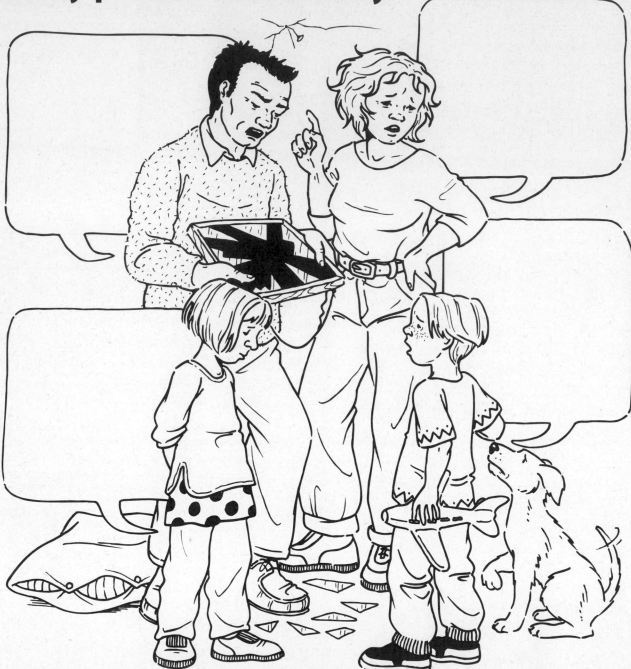

■ Consider these questions to help you fill in the speech bubbles.

1. What do you think has happened?
2. What is the mother feeling?
3. What is the father feeling?
4. Why do they have these feelings?
5. What are the children feeling?
6. Why do you think they are feeling this way?
7. What could the children do to make things better?
8. What could the parents say then?

Photocopiables

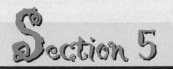

Section 5 — LEARN TO RESPECT THE DIFFERENCES BETWEEN PEOPLE

The activities in this section focus on children:
- generating an environment in which differences are respected
- listening to and accepting other points of view
- seeing the world from other people's perspectives
- recognizing worth in others
- questioning media images and stereotypes, different prejudices, discrimination and so on
- recognizing other social groups, such as people of a different age or culture.

'ISMS'

RESOURCES AND CLASSROOM ORGANIZATION

Prepare in advance the question and answer game cards from photocopiable pages 41 and 42, one set for each group of children. Number the cards on the reverse side, using red for questions and green for answers, and put each set into a polythene bag. You will also need: a dice and shaker; dictionaries.

Children play in groups of six (as two teams of three) and finish with a class discussion.

WHAT TO DO

Tell the children that they are going to study 'isms'! Sexism, racism… Ask: *What do we mean by, for example, racism?* If they don't know, ask them to look the word up in a dictionary. (It means discriminating against someone because of their race, believing that some races are superior to others, or being abusive or aggressive towards members of another race. Discrimination means the unfair treatment of a person, racial group or minority, for example.)

Divide the class into their groups, explaining that they are going to find out more by playing a game. Go through the following rules with the children.

Rules

1. The first player to throw a six starts the game.
2. Each player throws the dice in turn, takes the question card corresponding to the number shown and reads out the situation.
3. He or she, with help from team-mates if necessary, decides which 'ism' the situation shows, or what sort of discrimination against a particular person, and explains (with reasons) to the opposite team.
4. The opposite team discuss the answer, state whether they agree with it or not, and then check by reading out the appropriate answer card.
5. If the player was correct, his or her team keep both the question and answer cards; if wrong, the opposing team keeps them.
6. If there are no cards left corresponding to the number thrown on the dice, the player has up to two more turns before passing on the dice.
7. The game is continued until all the cards are used up.
8. The winning team is the one with the most cards.

When the groups have all finished the game, ask for their card totals and congratulate all those who did well. Ask each group to talk about one situation which they correctly explained during the game, and so open discussion on the meanings of racism, sexism, ageism, 'sizeism' and 'disabledism'!

OBJECTIVES

To enable children to:
- question media images and stereotypes
- recognize other social groups, for example by their culture or age
- learn skills for following instructions
- practise co-operative skills in a team situation
- listen to and accept other points of view.

CROSS-CURRICULAR LINKS

ENGLISH

Listening to others' reactions; taking turns in speaking; qualifying or justifying what they think after listening to other opinions and accounts; dealing politely with opposing points of view; dictionary work.

Ready to go! IDEAS FOR PSHE

Ask the children to imagine that they are someone described in one of the statements, for example the girl in the wheelchair. Ask: *How does it feel to be discriminated against?* (Unfair, upsetting, frustrating, humiliating.) *What can we do to make sure people are not discriminated against?* (Challenge discrimination when we find it, help people to make changes, help charities which support minority groups like those with limited hearing.)

Conclude by asking the children what they have learned and how this will affect their future thinking and actions.

Now or later

■ What other 'isms' can the children think of (for example, 'No pushchairs allowed'!)? Some 'isms' are for safety, such as people not being allowed to drink alcohol in a pub before the age of 18.

■ Invite a speaker who has personal experience of discrimination, or who works for a relevant charity (for example, Help the Aged), to come in to talk to the class.

■ Collect examples of action against discrimination (such as installation of ramps for wheelchairs) from the local paper, or as seen in the local area.

STEREOTYPES

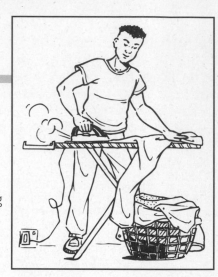

OBJECTIVES

To enable children to:
■ see the world from other people's perspectives
■ question media images and stereotypes.

CROSS-CURRICULAR LINKS

ENGLISH

Exploring, developing and explaining ideas; sharing ideas, insights and opinions; drama.

RESOURCES AND CLASSROOM ORGANIZATION

You will need a copy of photocopiable page 43 for each pair of children; an illustration or a photograph (A4 size) showing an image that is non-stereotypical, such as a man doing the ironing or making clothes using a sewing machine.

Class work is followed by work in pairs, and concludes with a whole-class discussion.

WHAT TO DO

Start by showing the class the picture and ask them if they think there is anything unusual about it. The picture goes against our idea of a stereotype, for example men or boys not doing the ironing! Ask: *What do we mean by a 'stereotype'?* (A stereotype is a standardized image or rigid idea of a type of person, and what he or she should or shouldn't do, say or wear, and so on. For example, 'all teenagers are tearaways', 'old people sit around all day', 'blond beautiful ladies are all bimbos [unintelligent]'.)

Give out copies of photocopiable page 43 and ask the children to look at the pictures, working in pairs. Encourage them to consider the pairs of pictures, discuss which is the stereotype and give their reasons.

Discussion points for the stereotypes on photocopiable page 43

The stereotypical woman stays at home and frets about how clean the washing is, or just does the household chores all the time. In fact, a lot of women go out to work, and most have interests other than housework!

The stereotypical old person is rather boring and doesn't do much at all! However, many older people are extremely active (running the London marathon, for example) and have very interesting lives.

The stereotypical teenager is noisy, doesn't think of others' feelings and is only interested in having fun. In fact, of course, there are many who are quiet, caring (and even studious!).

The stereotypical man is only interested in fast cars (and football and going to the pub). In reality, lots of men enjoy being with their families and caring for the children.

Ask for volunteers from the class to explain which stereotypes they have identified, and why. Ask: *Are stereotypes fair?* They are sometimes based on traditional views about what is the usual behaviour or attitude of men, women, boys and girls, old and young. *Should we be so rigid and restrictive in our thinking about what anyone can do or be?* For example, is there any good reason why boys and men should not do housework? It may be traditionally a woman's role because in the past, not so many women had full-time jobs, but now lots of women as well as men go out to work.

Ask: *What other examples of stereotyping can you think of?* Suggest that the children think about characters portrayed on television, in newspapers, magazines, comics and advertisements. An example might be male scientists in white coats giving advice about domestic appliances, or ever-smiling babies in pristine clothes. Sexual stereotyping shows women as weak, gentle, caring, domestic, and men as strong, aggressive and dominant. Can the children think of any examples where stereotypes are 'broken' on television or in real life?

Conclude by asking the children what they felt about this activity and how it might influence them in the future. Will they be more aware of the danger of stereotyping, and of making assumptions about what people can or cannot be or do?

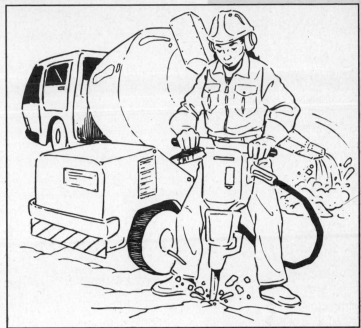

NOW OR LATER

■ Ask the children to cut out the pictures on the photocopiable sheet, glue them onto a sheet of paper and write about each one underneath.

■ Children could bring in articles and advertisements showing stereotyping, or the opposite, for discussion. These could then be displayed on a noticeboard with appropriate captions.

■ Small groups of children could each make up a drama which involves the questioning of someone who has 'broken' a stereotype, for example a male nurse or a female motor mechanic, asking the person what it feels like and whether they meet any prejudice.

■ Children could draw their own pictures of stereotypes!

■ Using non-fiction books or CD-ROMs, children could find out about the first woman MP, doctor or astronaut, in the UK or elsewhere.

WE AGREE TO DIFFER

RESOURCES AND CLASSROOM ORGANIZATION

Prepare in advance information about topic(s) to be debated. (Children could be asked to research information for homework.) Topics, expressed as 'the motion for debate', might include 'All firearms should be banned', 'We do/don't need a monarchy', 'City centres would be better without cars'. You will also need: a notebook for each child; writing materials.

The class is divided in half, and each half divided again to give 'for' and 'against' arguments. Children work in groups, then as half a class and conclude with a whole-class discussion.

WHAT TO DO

Divide the class into four groups (as above). Give each group the relevant information and tell them whether they are to be 'for' or 'against' the motion. Allow

OBJECTIVES

To enable children to:
■ generate an environment in which differences are respected
■ listen to and accept other points of view
■ see the world from other people's perspectives
■ distinguish between 'fact' and 'opinion'.

CROSS-CURRICULAR LINKS

ENGLISH

Communicating effectively in speech and writing; listening with understanding; formulating, clarifying and expressing ideas; responding appropriately to others; sharing insights, ideas and opinions; qualifying or justifying what they think after listening to others' opinions; dealing politely with other points of view.

them about 15 minutes to read and discuss it and make notes about key points. Each group may have a spokesperson, if wished, or several people may speak. Explain that in a debate you can argue for your side even if that is not what you actually believe. Points must be made politely! Make it clear that people must be allowed to have their say without heckling. Ask them to listen out for when a speaker is giving them a *fact*, or expressing an *opinion,* and to make notes on this. Check that all the children understand the difference between a fact and an opinion.

Now set up the debate. Explain that half the class will observe while the others debate. One side will propose the motion, for example 'This house believes that fox hunting should be banned', and argue their case. The opposition then replies using counter arguments. The whole class votes on whether the motion is carried or lost, and both the winners and losers get a round of applause. If time allows, let the other half of the class have their turn – or this can take place on a later occasion.

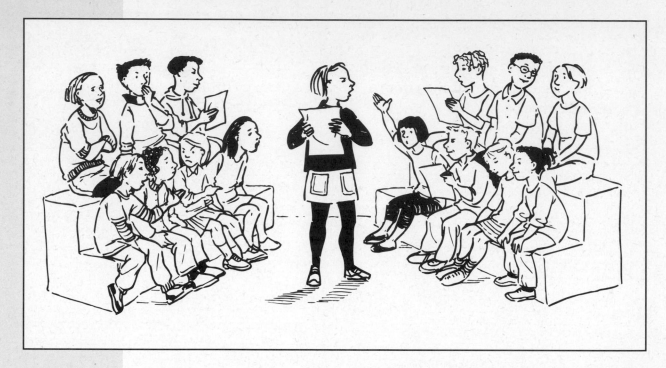

Afterwards ask the children how they felt about the activity. Hopefully it was interesting and fun even though it may have been frustrating at times! *Was it easy or difficult to express what you wanted to say? Is it important to listen to everyone's point of view?* (Yes, this is what we call democracy. Debates like this take place in parliament before a vote is taken.) Ask for examples of fact and opinion from the debate. What have they learned from the debate?

NOW OR LATER

■ With the proposed motion as the title, children could write out the main points from their debate under 'pros' and 'cons' headings, and end by explaining their opinions with reasons.

■ Children could observe a debate taking place at a debating society, the local council, or perhaps watch a video of a debate from the House of Commons.

■ Children could find out more about our democratic government and how it works. They could contact the Parliamentary Education Unit at:
Room 604, Norman Shaw Building (North), London SW1A 2TT, or on e-mail: edunit@parliament.uk. Look for the 'Explore Parliament' website by following links from www.parliament.uk.

■ The debate could be 'replayed' as a showpiece for an assembly or open day, with a narrator explaining the procedure and informing the audience about the nature of democracy.

■ A debating society could be set up at school, perhaps meeting once each half-term.

The 'isms' game – question cards

1. Smartly dressed Nicole has a job interview as a typist. The interviewer can't help noticing she is a very large woman. Although Nicole demonstrates fast, accurate typing skills, the job is given to a slower but slimmer candidate.

2. Paul and Suzy have moved into a new house. They invite all their neighbours to their housewarming party, except the old couple on the corner who they think would not enjoy a party.

3. A young blind man wishing to keep fit and healthy is turned away from a sports centre because dogs aren't allowed in the building.

4. A very tall man is in a clothing shop looking through racks of suits. An assistant approaches and says, "I'm afraid we don't stock giant sizes, Sir!"

5. Maria does exactly the same work as her colleague Max, but is paid less per hour then he is.

6. In a group of students interviewed for student training, Manjit Singh is easily the best qualified, but is the last to be offered a place on the scheme.

1a. Eric is a fit, pleasant and healthy 75-year-old. He offers his help as a driver to a local charity who have advertised for more people. He is turned down by them.

2a. Some of the crowd at a football match keep shouting, "Go back to Africa," each time a black player has the ball.

3a. A group of car mechanics threaten to go on strike because a woman has been appointed head of their team.

4a. A teenage girl in a wheelchair is unable to go with her friends to see the latest film because there are no ramps at her local cinema.

5a. Laura Biggs wants to join the local golf club, but is surprised to find that women are only allowed to play on Saturday mornings.

6a. An experienced, highly thought of male nurse is not selected for one of the few places on a midwifery course (to learn how to deliver babies) he applied for.

The 'isms' game – answer cards

1. **'Sizeism'.** The woman is discriminated against because she is very large.

2. **Ageism.** The couple are discriminated against because of their age (being old).

3. **'Disabledism'.** The man is discriminated against because of his disability.

4. **'Sizeism'.** The man is discriminated against (being treated badly) because he is so tall.

5. **Sexism.** The woman is discriminated against because of her sex (being female).

6. **Racism.** The man is discriminated against because of his race.

1a. **Ageism.** The man is discriminated against because of his age (being old).

2a. **Racism.** The man is being treated abusively because of his race.

3a. **Sexism.** The woman is being treated badly because of her sex (being female).

4a. **'Disabledism'.** The girl is being discriminated against because of her disability.

5a. **Sexism.** The woman is being discriminated against because of her sex (being female).

6a. **Sexism.** The man is being discriminated against because of his sex (being male).

Stereotype pairs

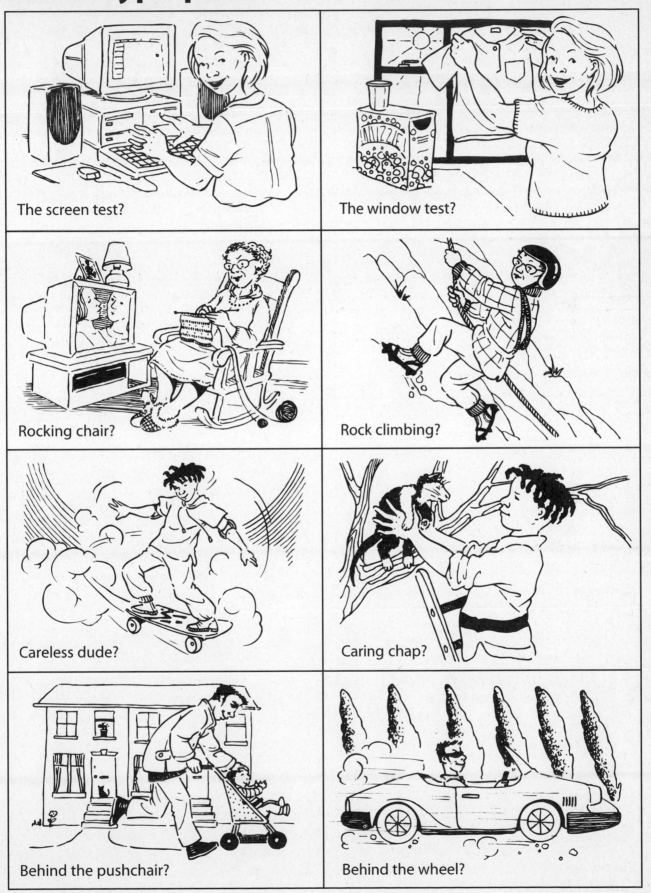

The screen test?

The window test?

Rocking chair?

Rock climbing?

Careless dude?

Caring chap?

Behind the pushchair?

Behind the wheel?

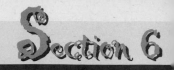
The activities in this section focus on children:
- facing challenges in a supportive environment
- taking responsibility for themselves, including their behaviour
- being involved in the development and implementation of an anti-bullying policy
- looking ahead, for example to growing up, the transition to secondary school
- developing trust and reliability.

ZERO TOLERANCE!

OBJECTIVES

To enable children to:
- face challenges in a supportive environment
- take responsibility for their own behaviour
- be involved in the development and implementation of an anti-bullying policy.

CROSS-CURRICULAR LINKS

ENGLISH

Sharing ideas, insights and opinions; qualifying or justifying what they think; reading; writing.

ICT

Using equipment for a variety of purposes.

ART

Expressing ideas.

DESIGN & TECHNOLOGY

Using information sources for designing; considering the purpose of a design.

RESOURCES AND CLASSROOM ORGANIZATION

You will need a copy of photocopiable page 50 and paper for each small group; flip chart or board; writing materials.

Children work in small groups who share their findings for class discussion.

WHAT TO DO

Suggest to the class that it might be appropriate from time to time to reconsider relationships within the school and class, and particularly to focus on the issue of bullying. How well do they feel this is (or isn't) being controlled? Bullying can happen in many situations throughout life, so we all need to be aware of it and be confident that we know what to do if we are ever victims, and who we can ask for help.

Ask the children, working in their small groups, to discuss a definition of bullying: *What exactly is bullying?* and then to write down their ideas. Make sure that all the children are aware that bullying is when a person, or group of people, is being *deliberately* unkind to an individual or other group, calling them names, taking their things away or physically hurting them. Words and labels *do* hurt.

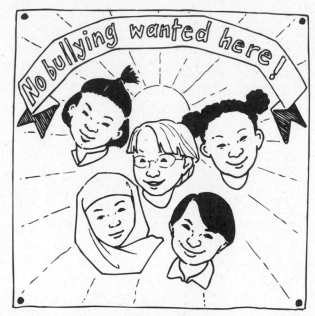

Collect in their ideas and write them on the flip chart, explaining that some bullying can be very subtle and is often excused as only being meant as a joke. Explain that things 'just meant as a joke' are *not* a joke if the person won't stop when asked.

Now, using photocopiable page 50, explain that each group is going to discuss three areas:
- what an individual can do if bullied (the 'sun' questions)
- how the bullies themselves might be helped to change (the 'star' questions)
- what the school can do (the 'moon' questions).

Give the small groups their photocopiable sheets, to stimulate discussion, and some paper for them to make notes. Following this, ask each group to tell the class their conclusions, giving their reasons for one or two issues. Formulate the class or school anti-bullying policy by writing up key statements on the flip chart.

Finally, discuss what action needs to be taken for the whole school to become involved (see 'Now or later'). Ask: *What can each of us do to make sure that bullying does not occur at our school in the future?*

NOW OR LATER

■ Children could design anti-bullying posters to be put up around the school. Discuss effective posters – bold clear lettering, limited writing, eye-catching effects and so on (text could include 'Our school says NO! to bullying', 'Bully off').

■ Ask the children to design, illustrate and print out the school's anti-bullying policy and arrange for every child to receive a copy.

■ For other ideas, see 'What would you like your school to do?' on photocopiable page 50.

■ Children could contact Kidscape, 2 Grosvenor Gardens, London SW1W 0DH, to ask for their 'Bullying' or 'Child Protection' packs, enclosing an A4 self-addressed envelope with a 60p stamp.

CARING FOR OTHERS

RESOURCES AND CLASSROOM ORGANIZATION

Set up visits over several days or weeks with a Reception or Year 1 class. You will need: a Reception or Year 1 level book; notebooks for all the children, materials for book-making (white and coloured card, fabrics, paper, scissors, felt-tipped pens and so on); rough paper; writing materials.

Before and after making books in pairs or small groups, the children work in small groups with younger children, and take part in a final class analysis of the activity.

WHAT TO DO

Start by showing a Reception or Year 1 level book to the class and reading it out loud. Ask the children if they think it is a suitable book for *them*. (Obviously not, as it was designed for young children!) Discuss the features of the book – clear bright pictures, limited vocabulary and a simple story, for example.

Explain to the children that they are going to become authors and make books for a class of younger children (tell them which class it is). First they will need to do some research to find out the interests and capabilities of the children for whom they are writing. Discuss what they will need to find out and make a list of important points such as the children's reading levels, their attention spans, and so on.

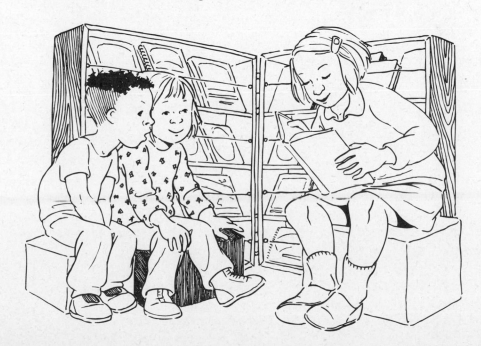

OBJECTIVES

To enable children to:
■ learn to care for other people
■ think about the needs of other people
■ learn to become responsible
■ develop trust and reliability.

CROSS-CURRICULAR LINKS

ENGLISH

Listening and responding to a range of people; expressing themselves confidently and clearly; writing for varied purposes, in response to a variety of stimuli.

DESIGN & TECHNOLOGY

Using information sources to help in designing; generating ideas and considering the purpose of a design; evaluating design ideas and improving them.

ART

Expressing ideas and feelings; recording what has been experienced, observed and imagined.

Take the children (a small group at a time, each child with a notebook) on a preliminary visit during the Reception (or Year 1) class's 'free play' time. Let them question the young children, talking and playing with them as well as reading books with them. Encourage the group to make notes on what they observe.

Return to your own classroom and discuss the children's findings and ideas. In the book that is going to be written, they will need to consider the storyline, vocabulary, length and details such as how large to make the writing. Have they thought about whether the book is going to be for young children to read, or is it to be read to them? How can they make the book exciting? Discuss ideas such as using peepholes, flaps, pop-up sections and sparkly, shiny, textured materials.

The children should now plan their books on rough paper, deciding on the cover, title page, contents page (if appropriate), page layout and illustrations, and with your approval progress to make the real thing.

When the books are completed, arrange for the class to visit the Reception (or Year 1) class to read the stories in small groups, noting children's responses carefully. The session should end with mutual thanks and appreciation!

Conclude with a debriefing session, once you have returned to your own classroom. Questions to ask might include: *Did the children enjoy your book? Did they like a particular part especially, and if so why do you think this was? Did anything not go quite according to plan, and if not, why do you think this was? How might you improve on your book design in the future? How did you feel about reading to the younger children? Would you like to do this again? What do you think younger children gain by listening to stories being read to them? What did you gain from the experience? How do you think you might use this in the future – as a babysitter, a parent or an aunt/uncle?*

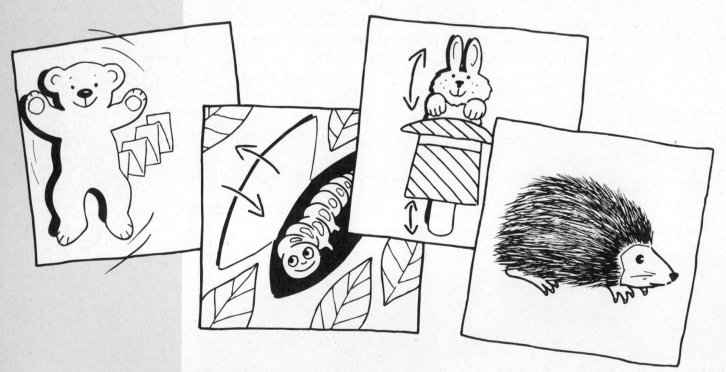

NOW OR LATER

■ Children could 'write up' their activity, explaining the stages of the process of producing their book, commenting on its success and any changes to be made.

■ Expand the theme to consider books for babies, and what the specifications might be – such as the product should be safe to be put into the mouth!

■ Groups could consider what criteria to use when designing an educational toy, or number game, for younger children.

■ Let the children compare themselves with the younger children in terms of their capabilities, maturity, book choices and so on.

■ In consultation with the Reception (or Year 1) teacher, the class could design and make a Big Book to be used during the Literacy Hour.

WHAT WOULD YOU DO?

RESOURCES AND CLASSROOM ORGANIZATION

You will need: board or flip chart; paper; writing materials.

After a class introduction, children work in groups, then share their ideas in a final class discussion.

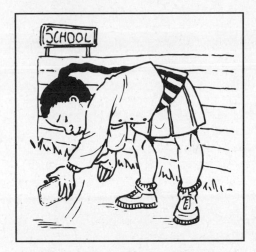

WHAT TO DO

Start by saying to the class: *Supposing you had come across a purse full of money this morning on your way to school, what would you have done?* Talk briefly about why it would have been wrong to keep it. How would they have felt if they had lost their own purse and it was returned, or alternatively, never found? *Why would it have been right to hand it in at school?* (This would have meant that there would have been a chance of it being returned it to its owner, perhaps after first having been passed to the police.) Explain that the way people behave in these situations depends on their moral values – their belief in right and wrong.

Now divide the children into small groups of three or four and give out some paper to each group. Explain that they are going to discuss the purse incident and three others. These are:

■ You have noticed that a four-year-old child is quietly removing all the free gifts from the comics and magazines in a newsagents, and pocketing them (his mother is engrossed in a magazine that she is reading and isn't aware of the situation – nor is the shop assistant).
■ You see two nine-year-olds throwing stones at the windows of an empty house.
■ Sitting on a park bench, you see a teenage girl throw a crisp packet on the ground as she walks along the path, eating snacks.

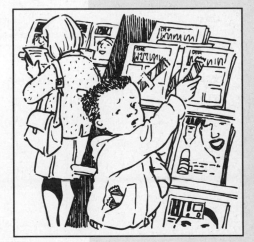

Write the situations on the board, including the 'purse' one already discussed as the fourth situation. Ask the children to write notes on every aspect they can think of for the four situations, and be ready to present their ideas of what would be 'right' and 'wrong' to the class. Depending on the ability of the children, the following points might be raised before or after the group discussions:

■ *Situation 1:* Should you tell the child yourself that it's wrong and make him or her put back the gifts, or tell the parent (who hasn't noticed) or the shop assistant? Is a child as young as four able to tell the difference between right and wrong? He or she

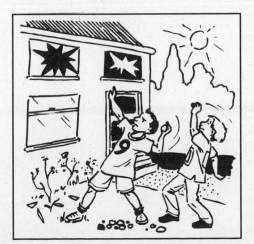

may not realize that it is stealing. Who do the 'free' gifts actually belong to? How could you explain this to the child? Are there other issues here? (For example, good parenting!)
■ *Situation 2:* Why do you think the children are throwing stones? Does it matter if damage is caused as the house is empty anyway? Who would have to pay for the repairs? What is the name for deliberate damage to property like this? Would it be safe to try and stop the children yourself? Should the police be informed straight away, or the parents first, if you know them? Are

OBJECTIVES
To enable children to:
■ take responsibility for themselves, including their behaviour
■ face challenges in a supportive environment
■ develop trust and reliability
■ consider moral values.

CROSS-CURRICULAR LINKS
ENGLISH
Formulating, clarifying and expressing ideas; predicting outcomes; discussing possibilities; giving reasons for opinions; listening to others' reactions; dealing politely with opposing points of view; using the conventions of discussion, for example taking turns in speaking; drama – role-play.

the children old enough to know what they are doing? Is their safety at risk? Who is responsible for the children's actions?

■ *Situation 3:* Why do you think the girl just threw away the packet? Does throwing a bit of litter on the ground really matter? After all, people are employed to clean up the streets anyway! What does our environment look like littered with rubbish? Who pays the street-cleaners' wages? Should you confront the girl yourself or just put the litter in a bin?

■ *Situation 4:* See the questions used at the beginning of 'What to do'.

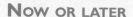

End by helping the children to summarize what they have discussed about moral values – what they believe is right and wrong.

NOW OR LATER

■ Children could role-play the given situations in small groups, adding characters such as parents and policemen/women and experimenting with different outcomes. The class as the audience could question each character to see how they are feeling about the situation.

■ Ask the children to draw pictures of themselves, each one with a different speech bubble that gives one reason why they would not throw stones at windows, drop litter and so on.

■ Can the children think of their own moral dilemmas? Encourage them to hold mini-debates to discuss what to do about them.

■ Children could find out more about morals and ethics, and what is meant by a 'philosophy of life' .

EXPECTATIONS OF SECONDARY SCHOOL

OBJECTIVES

To enable children to:
■ face challenges in a supportive environment
■ look ahead to the transition to secondary school
■ have confidence about the near future
■ become more independent
■ take responsibility for themselves including their behaviour.

CROSS-CURRICULAR LINKS

ENGLISH
Planning, predicting, investigating, reporting and re-presenting information in different forms.

GEOGRAPHY
Studying the locality.

ICT
Using equipment to carry out a variety of functions.

RESOURCES AND CLASSROOM ORGANIZATION

You will need: a local map, cassette players with microphones and cassettes; pictures of the local secondary schools that most children will be going to; large sheets of paper for each group; board or flip chart; writing materials.

Divided into groups, children have a preparatory lesson, find out more for homework, then have a second lesson that involves reporting back.

WHAT TO DO

Display the pictures of the secondary schools and say: *Many of you will be thinking ahead to a few months' time when you will be going to secondary school. What do you think are the differences between primary and secondary schools?* As the children make suggestions, write them on the board. These might include: secondary school is usually a larger size; the children may have further to go (perhaps by bus) to get to school; they will have different teachers for different subjects; 'canteen' type lunches; more homework. *Are there any other changes you can think of?* (Perhaps making new friends; having a form tutor; being the youngest instead of the oldest in the school; having to be well organized, making sure that you take necessary items to school such as PE equipment.)

Explain that they will be making a visit to their new school later, to meet their new teachers. Starting at secondary school is one of the big changes we all have to make. Most people feel a little apprehensive about it, even if they don't show it! As with all new situations, we can help ourselves by finding out as much as we can in advance about what it will be like, and who will help us get used to things.

Ask the children to discuss all the things they would like to know about their new school and list everything on their sheets, working in their groups. For example, their lists may include the exact location, school hours, the uniform, how much homework they can expect to be given, sports, clubs and societies they can join, meal arrangements and how they will travel to the school.

Next, ask the groups to display their lists, and work as a class to decide how they can best get specific information – for example, from the school brochure or Internet website; by asking former pupils to come and answer questions about their experiences; by taping interviews with older brothers or sisters already at the secondary school (the class can decide what questions it would like to ask); by preparing a list of questions they would like answered when they visit the new school; by using street maps and bus or train timetables.

Make a class decision on which method pairs or small groups are going to use to obtain the required information on any one school, and agree on a date when this can be presented to the rest of the class.

Organize a second session with groups of children reporting about a particular school. If liked, one child per group could write the information on a large sheet of paper with the name and picture of the school at the top. Or the information could be printed out by computer as a fact sheet.

Summarize by asking what the children have learned. How did they feel about this activity? Are they happier now about their impending move to secondary school, and are they confident about finding information by different methods? Which was the most successful? Which allowed feelings as well as facts to be discussed?

NOW OR LATER

■ Put up a display about the secondary schools, using the map as a centrepiece. Place threads onto the map which lead out from the schools to information about them. Information could include pictures of a boy and girl wearing the school uniform, how most children get to the school, the name and photograph of the headteacher, the number of pupils there, the names of past pupils who go there, and so on.

■ Invite a guest from a local secondary school – for example the primary school liaison teacher, or even an older ex-pupil – to come and talk to the children about the transition to secondary school.

■ Ask children who have made visits to their proposed secondary schools to write about their experiences and share them with the class.

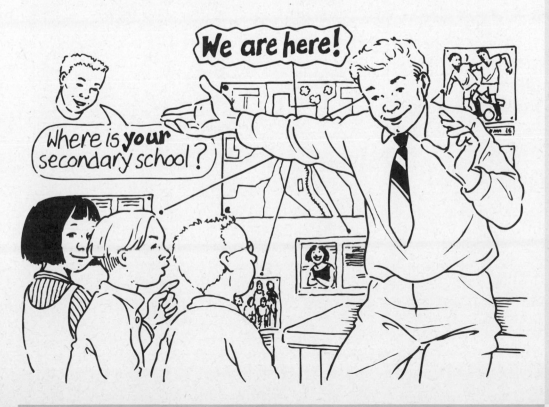

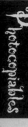
Photocopiables

Name   Date

What can we do about bullying?

If you are being bullied…

Tell an adult straight away – who? Talk to a friend too?

No one deserves to be bullied. Is this true?

It is *not* your fault if you are being bullied. True?

If you are being bullied

If you don't tell anyone, no one can help you. True?

Be assertive. Tell the bully "No" firmly and walk away. Could this work?

Work out a reply to the bully? For example, repeat what they say, make a joke or say, "What's your problem?"

Try not to show it if you are upset, and don't fight back. Why not?

Nobody likes bullies (people may *pretend* to – why?).

Bullies need help to change. True? Who could they go to?

What about the bullies? Do we need to think about them?

Why do you think some people bully others?

Do you think bullies are happy people?

■ Discuss each statement and make notes.

Help every class to discuss bullying and put forward their ideas.

Find out more information, for example from Kidscape.

Have anti-bullying assemblies.

What would you like your school to do?

Have anti-bullying posters around the school.

Invite a speaker to tell everyone more about bullying.

All staff discuss bullying and agree a policy.

Have a box where pupils can put a note about bullying.

Have a special adult or child trained to help bullying victims.

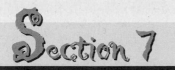
LEARN TO BECOME GOOD CITIZENS

The activities in this section focus on children:
■ understanding and appreciating the communities to which they belong locally, nationally and internationally
■ taking a responsible role in school
■ appreciating the impact that human activity has on animals and the environment
■ learning about treating animals with care and sensitivity
■ understanding how they and others can cause changes for the better (or worse) in the wider community
■ developing a concern for communities where human needs are not always met
■ developing a sense of fair play.

SOCIETY MATTERS

RESOURCES AND CLASSROOM ORGANIZATION

You will need: a copy of photocopiable page 56 and a large sheet of paper for each group; writing materials.

After a whole-class introductory session, the children work in groups. This is followed by a class discussion.

WHAT TO DO

Explain to the class that they are going to be considering what people mean when they talk about 'society'. What 'societies' have they heard of? Perhaps they have heard of drama and music societies, angling societies, the Royal Society for the Protection of Birds, and so on. These are all groups of people who join together for a particular shared activity.

Now explain that there is another meaning for society, namely, the 'society' that we live in all the time. Our school is a small version of such a society, where people, working together, agree to behave in certain acceptable ways, and believe in the same things. Ask: *How have we all agreed to behave?* (Be polite, keep to the school rules, be kind to each other, and so on.) *What sorts of things do we believe in?* (The value of work and education, in raising money for charities, helping others who are less well off than ourselves and looking after younger children.) *Who and what do we need to enable us to do these things?* (Teachers, assistants, caretakers, secretaries – all have their role in this society, and we also need buildings, classrooms, tables, desks, playgrounds, kitchens and so on.) The physical things are called the 'infrastructure' of a society.

OBJECTIVES
To enable children to:
■ understand the structure of a society
■ appreciate the value of being part of a society
■ appreciate school values
■ take a responsible role in school.

CROSS-CURRICULAR LINKS
ENGLISH
Exploring, developing and explaining ideas; writing in response to a wide range of stimuli.

GEOGRAPHY
Developing knowledge of human settlements and the supply of goods.

HISTORY
Understanding ancient civilization; learning about the past from a range of sources.

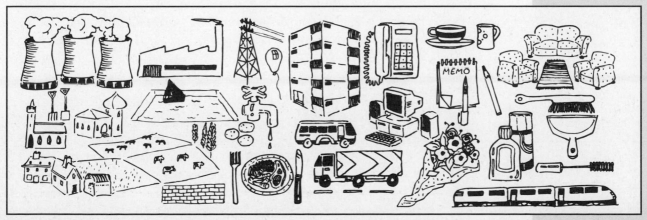

Next, divide the class into small groups, giving each group a copy of photocopiable page 56 and a large sheet of paper. Read out the introductory text and explain the questions if necessary. Ask the children to discuss each question and write their answers on the large sheet. Give them half an hour to complete the task.

Now with the whole class consider each of the three questions in turn, asking the groups for their contributions under the headings 'First', 'Later' and 'Long term'. Help them to the following understanding:

■ A 'society' means people who are living together in a community. It has organizations that provide different services to the community (such as health care). There are many different relationships and interactions between the organizations and between individuals.

■ 'Services' include local and national government, financial, health, defence/armed forces, emergency, law and order, water boards, farming, communication systems, transport, education, culture, arts, entertainment, tourism/holidays, religions, charities, construction, engineering, architectural, scientific research, service industries, leisure, health and fitness, and social services.

■ 'Infrastructures' are the roads, railways, buildings, transmitters, electricity pylons, gas and water pipes, lampposts, pavements and so on which allow the services to function properly.

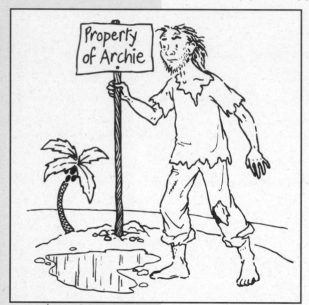

■ An individual person would not be able to provide all the services listed for him or herself, and so depends on and benefits from society for most things. In our country we have a 'high standard of living' because of our very complex society.

■ Contributions to society by children might include being a pleasant, responsible citizen (!), respecting the local environment, helping needy people and charities. In the future, having a job and paying taxes makes a contribution to society.

Afterwards, discuss each group's choices, encouraging them to 'argue their case' by explaining their reasons for their chosen priorities.

Point out that with their immediate, medium and long term plans they have actually repeated the historical process which our 'western' society has gone through (from primitive cave dwelling to the complex structures of today).

Finally, ask the children to consider what life might be like for the shipwrecked people *without* any organized society. There might be fighting over scarce resources such as a water supply. Everyone would have to do everything for themselves instead of helping each other and sharing their skills.

So can they now see what the benefits of a society are for the individual? On their own, individuals cannot do very much for themselves, but if everyone contributes, we can all benefit from each other's skills. What have they learned? Will this help them to be good citizens in the future?

NOW OR LATER

■ Develop the theme further by dividing the class into groups to consider in more detail how they would organize the following areas of their island society: transport, food, education, health and social services, government (and other areas such as religious/spiritual life, defence, energy supply, communications, and so on). Ask the groups to present their findings to the class for discussion.

■ Ask the children to think more about their own school as a mini-society. How can each individual contribute? Ideas may range from being well behaved to helping the school (for example by manning a telephone at lunchtime) or by taking part in the decision-making process of the school (such as in a school council).

■ Children could find out more about their local community and its needs, and how they could become involved in meeting these (for example, by inviting senior citizens to a school performance or volunteering for litter collection in the local park).

WHO CARES ABOUT ANIMALS?

RESOURCES AND CLASSROOM ORGANIZATION

Organize some weeks in advance for groups of children to choose an animal topic and prepare a talk on it after carrying out some research. They should choose from:

■ animals in circuses or in zoos – the pros and cons in each case
■ commercial fishing methods and dolphin-friendly tuna fishing
■ battery versus free-range hens in the production of eggs
■ the work of the RSPCA, and what is meant by their 'Freedom Food' label
■ the organization Compassion in World Farming and their campaigns, for example against the exporting of live animals
■ the work of the World Wide Fund for Nature, and the protection of animals in danger of extinction.

You will also need: a flip chart, board or OHP; paper and writing materials.

Children work first in groups, then make their presentations to the class, continue with individual work and finish with a class discussion.

WHAT TO DO

Divide the class into groups and let them select the research topics they are interested in. Discuss how and where they will find the information, for example from the school or local library, CD-ROMs, the Internet, or by sending off for information from the relevant charities (see addresses in 'Now or later').

Ask each group to prepare a ten-minute talk with 'visual aids' – pictures, posters, drawings or OHTs. They should first discuss how each person in the group can contribute to the research and the presentation. For example, volunteer group members could each research a different aspect of the topic, and share their notes. Others could produce the illustrations. The group will need to decide who is to be the speaker and who will show the visual aids during the presentation.

Groups' presentations could be over several days. After each presentation, the group can be congratulated on any especially good aspects, and asked how easy or hard it was to get the information.

When all the groups have presented their findings, ask each child to jot down answers to a selection of the following questions:

■ *In what ways do you think animals are being mistreated?* (Farm animals reared in over-intensive conditions, with not enough room to exercise; dolphins caught in fishing nets; animals in cramped, boring conditions in zoos; pets being incorrectly looked after or being treated cruelly; wild animals losing their habitats or being hunted by man.)

■ *What is being done about this?* Mention the groups and campaigns talked about.

■ *Do you think enough is being done?*

■ *Do you think it is right that some humans seem to treat animals in any way they like?* (These are people who are not thinking about the fact that animals have rights and can feel pain, distress and boredom, in the same way that humans can; we should look after them in the best conditions possible.)

■ *Do we all have a responsibility for animal welfare?*

■ *What could we as a class do to try to make sure that as many animals as possible are fairly treated?* (Those with pets can make sure they know how to look after them

OBJECTIVES

To enable children to:
■ appreciate the impact that human activity has on animals and the environment
■ think about the needs of animals
■ learn to care about animals
■ understand how they and others can cause changes for the better, or worse, in the wider community
■ learn to do some research by themselves
■ practise speaking confidently in front of an audience.

CROSS-CURRICULAR LINKS

ENGLISH

Exploring, developing and explaining ideas; expressing themselves confidently and clearly; reading for information; writing in response to a range of stimuli.

correctly. The class and individuals can choose to support charities concerned with animal welfare.)

To conclude the activity, discuss the children's answers and ask them if they would like to find out more about any particular issue.

NOW OR LATER

■ Children could consider the issue of meat-eating versus vegetarianism.
■ The class could adopt and raise money for a specific charity and invite a representative to come and talk to them.
■ Children could collect further examples of organizations protecting or saving animals.
■ Some useful addresses include:

Freedom Food Ltd, The Manor House, Causeway, Horsham, West Sussex RH12 1HG

RSPCA Education, RSPCA HQ, Causeway, Horsham, West Sussex RH12 1HG

Compassion in World Farming Trust (CIWFT), Charles House, 5A Charles Street, Petersfield, Hants GU32 3EH

CIWF Ireland at: CIWF, Salmon Weir, Hanover Street, Cork, Ireland

World Wide Fund for Nature (WWF–UK), Panda House, Weyside Park, Godalming, Surrey GU7 1XR.

FAIR TRADE FOR ALL

OBJECTIVES

To enable children to:
■ develop a concern for communities where human needs are not always met
■ begin to take on a wider sense of social responsibility
■ understand how they and others can cause changes for better or worse in the wider community
■ develop a sense of fairness.

CROSS-CURRICULAR LINKS

ENGLISH

Sharing ideas, insights and opinions; reading for information; dictionary work.

GEOGRAPHY

Understanding about the supply of goods; gaining awareness of the global positions of various countries.

ICT

Using equipment as a research tool and for a variety of other functions.

RESOURCES AND CLASSROOM ORGANIZATION

You will need: a copy of photocopiable page 57 for each pair of children; writing materials.

Children work as a whole class, then in pairs and fours, followed by a final class discussion.

WHAT TO DO

Explain to the children that they are going to be thinking about the poorer countries in the world, and how we can trade fairly with them to enable them to work their way successfully out of poverty. Read out the following (or use your own words to explain).

> In this country we live in what is called the 'developed world'. We have education, medical care, many industries and services, and most people have enough food, shelter, warmth and other basic necessities. We are relatively rich and have a high standard of living. Many countries (some in Africa, Asia and Latin America, for example) compared with us are very poor. They are referred to as 'developing' countries (or sometimes as 'third world' countries). Many of their people do not have enough to eat, or even clean water to drink. To make matters worse, they are often exploited (that is, used unfairly) by the richer nations. Countries like ours sometimes do not pay a fair price for the food and goods they buy from third world countries, so although their people work extremely hard, they never have enough money to look after their families properly.

Check that the children understand the meaning of 'exploited', 'developed', 'trade' and so on.

Ask the children to work in pairs and imagine that they own a rich, but responsible, company in this country with a chain of supermarkets – called... (let them make up their own company name). Their supermarket chain wants to buy coffee, tea or cocoa from a Central American or African country. Give each pair a copy of photocopiable page 57 and ask them to read and discuss it. They must decide which statements to put in their fair trade policy. Ask: *What does a 'policy'*

Answers to 'Our policy is fair trade!' on photocopiable page 57

The fair practice statements are 1, 3, 5, 7, 9 and 12.

The unfair statements are 2, 4, 6, 8, 10 and 11.

mean? (What someone has decided to do.) Which practices will their company choose and why? Ask the pairs to join into fours and discuss their findings, then read out the correct answers for everyone to check. Point out that the unfair practices do go on today in companies that are exploiting developing countries.

End with a class discussion about fair trade issues. Can they explain *why* unfair practices are unfair? What would it feel like to be a worker in a poor country who has to work under these conditions of uncertainty? Mention that there is an international organization called 'Traidcraft' which is encouraging trade based on the fair trade practices they have been discussing, and is against 'exploitation'. Some shops sell Traidcraft and other fair trade products, for example gifts, crafts, clothes, cards and foodstuffs, and these can also be ordered from a catalogue. Other organizations practising fair trade policies include 'Café Direct' and 'Clipper Teas'. (See 'Now or later'.)

Did the children realize that exploitation goes on? What else have they discovered? How can the children help to encourage fair trading in the future? Can they find local shops that sell fair trade products?

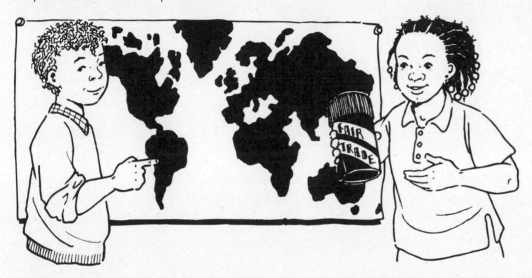

NOW OR LATER

■ Ask the children to clarify the definitions of the following words and write them down: developed country, developing country, trade, exploitation, goods, guaranteed, minimum, plantation.

■ Children could contact Traidcraft for leaflets to find out more about fair trade policy; they could ask for a catalogue and an order form for a game called 'Marketplace' (for six- to eleven-year-olds) – 12 to 36 children can play, and it would give them 'hands on' experience of what it feels like to trade and receive benefits for their community. The address is: Traidcraft PLC, Kingsway, Gateshead, Tyne and Wear NE11 0NE.

■ Children could do some research using books, CD-ROMs or the Internet to obtain more information about a developing country, and which crops they grow.

■ Using a world map, children could identify the countries the fair trade products come from, as well as other countries which grow coffee, tea and cocoa.

■ Ask the children to write a story about the life of a girl called Akasuwa and her family who work for a small company producing cocoa, before and after the company was helped by a fair trade organization.

■ Children could find out about the Office for Fair Trading.

■ Children could find out more about Clipper Teas on their Internet site – www.clipper-teas.com and Café Direct on www.cafedirect.co.uk.

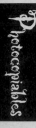
Photocopiables

Name _____   Date _____

Shipwrecked!

Imagine that you are part of a group of 50 people of all ages who have just been shipwrecked on an uninhabited island. The climate is quite like ours.
There is no chance of being rescued for years and years!

■ Discuss what your group would have to do to organize a 'society' where people could live together safely and happily. Look at the ideas below and decide:
1. which things you would do **first** (in the first day or few days)
2. which things you would do **later** (after a few weeks or months).

■ Write them down under **First** and **Later** headings on your paper, adding your own ideas.

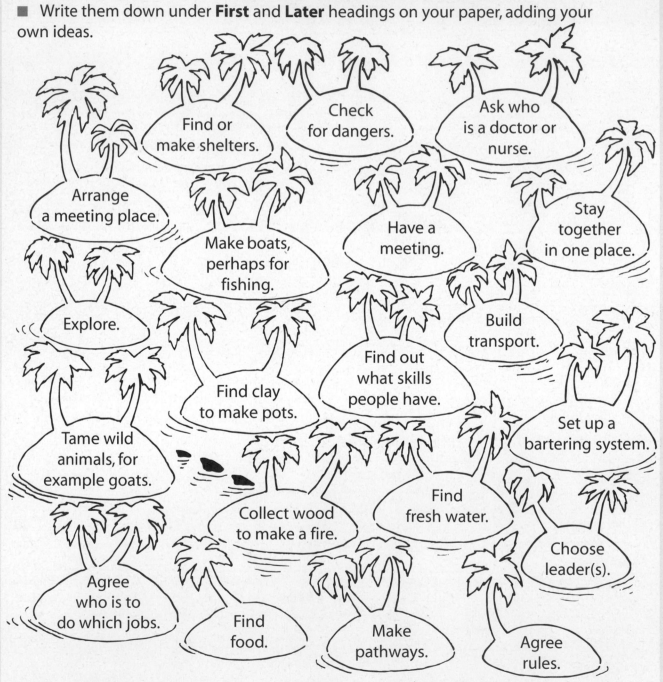

Find or make shelters.

Check for dangers.

Ask who is a doctor or nurse.

Arrange a meeting place.

Make boats, perhaps for fishing.

Have a meeting.

Stay together in one place.

Explore.

Build transport.

Find clay to make pots.

Find out what skills people have.

Set up a bartering system.

Tame wild animals, for example goats.

Collect wood to make a fire.

Find fresh water.

Choose leader(s).

Agree who is to do which jobs.

Find food.

Make pathways.

Agree rules.

■ Now think about what things you would do in the **long term** (over the years) and write them down, too. To help you, think of all the things we have in our society today.

Our policy is fair trade!

The name of our fair trade supermarket is:

■ Read the statements carefully first.
Highlight all the statements your supermarket will put in its fair trade policy.

1. We only trade with producers who provide **good conditions** for their workers, for example enough rest breaks and meal times.

2. The **long hours** worked by the crop-pickers do not concern us – it is up to the plantation owner to decide these.

3. We will pay a **guaranteed minimum** price directly to the workers.

4. We have the right to suddenly **drop** the **price** we pay (if our sales are low).

5. We will **pay** for orders **in advance** so workers do not have to owe money (be in debt) to buy equipment.

6. We **pay** the **landowner** and let him or her decide how much to pay the actual workers (which may not be enough).

7. We will encourage the use of **better equipment** and methods of crop-growing, for example, by giving expert help.

8. We do not worry about paying on time. **Payment** may sometimes be **delayed** long after we have received the goods.

9. We will work to develop a long-term relationship of **partnership** and co-operation with the workers.

10. Our only consideration is buying at the **cheapest** price possible.

11. We have the right to **cancel** our **orders** at any time with no warning or explanation.

12. We will help the workers to get **disease-resistant plants** which will give more reliable crops.

Photocopiables

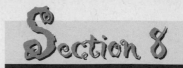
The activities in this section focus on children:
- making choices about their future
- being involved in assessing their work and setting targets for improvement
- developing key skills relevant to learning and work
- gaining experience and understanding of the world of work
- recognizing what they are good at and making choices
- interviewing adults, talking to adults and listening to adult experiences
- knowing it's OK to make mistakes and being able to learn from them.

PERSONAL ASSESSMENT

OBJECTIVES

To enable children to:
- reflect on their personal abilities and any weaknesses
- be involved in assessing their work
- use this assessment to help set targets for improvement.

CROSS-CURRICULAR LINKS

ENGLISH
Reading; exploring ideas; writing.

ICT
Using equipment for a variety of functions.

RESOURCES AND CLASSROOM ORGANIZATION

You will need: a copy of photocopiable page 62 for each child; writing materials. Children work individually, and also with you, at a one-to-one level.

WHAT TO DO

Give out the self-assessment sheets and let the children have a quick look at them. Explain that they will soon be completing them, but first of all, can they tell you why it is a good idea to think about *self*-assessment? It gives us all a chance to analyse and reflect on our abilities and skills. We can assess how much we have achieved, and what we would like to improve on for ourselves rather than have someone else point out these things to us.

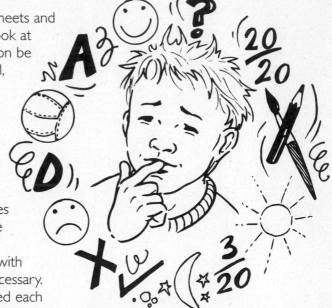

Go through the statements with the children, clarifying any if necessary. When each child has completed each section of the table, they should discuss it with you and receive praise for their achievements, and encouragement and support for suggested improvements. They should then fill in the 'I am especially proud of…' and 'I would like to improve…' sections.

When everyone has finished, ask the class how they felt about doing this activity. Has anyone discovered something about themselves that they hadn't realized before? How are they going to use their self-knowledge and understanding to help them in the future?

NOW OR LATER

- Children could write about their areas for improvement in more detail (perhaps using a computer and printed onto special paper) in the form of a pledge, 'I promise to do my best to improve…', to be signed by themselves and the teacher. This can then be reviewed regularly and praise given for any progress.
- Personal assessment sheets or resulting certificates of achievement could be presented at an assembly or special ceremony.
- Children could formulate a motto – 'Build on your strengths, strengthen your weaknesses!' or 'Progress through self-awareness'.

TELL ME ABOUT YOUR JOB

RESOURCES AND CLASSROOM ORGANIZATION

You will need: a board or flip chart; rough paper for each group; writing materials.

Children work in groups, followed by a class discussion, then in groups working on computers. The children interview adults and present their findings to the class.

WHAT TO DO

During this activity you will obviously need to be sensitive to children whose families are out of work.

Explain to the children that they are going to find out about the jobs (work) that people do. First ask: *Why do adults go out to work?* (Obviously to earn money to support themselves and their families, but hopefully also because they enjoy their work, and it gives them a role/status in society. Some people choose to do voluntary work, without pay, because they believe in the organization they are helping.)

Ask the children to form into small groups to consider the questions they would like to ask about someone's job or voluntary work. Explain that they will be actually using these to interview a friend or relative later on.

After about 15 minutes, get together as a class to share ideas about questions such as:
- What is your job title?
- What do you do in your job?
- What are the main skills that you have to use?
- What qualifications do you need for your job, and how did you get them?
- How do you get to work?
- How far away is your workplace?
- What hours do you work?
- Do you have problems with this or any other aspect of your work?
- What do you have to wear?
- Is a uniform (or equipment) provided, or do you have to purchase it?
- What do you enjoy most about your job, and why?
- What do you least enjoy about your job, and why?
- Would you recommend your job?

Following the discussion, ask the children to work in their groups to produce their list in the form of a questionnaire on the computer, and print out one copy for each child in the group. Children can take home their questionnaire and use it to interview someone about their job. If they don't have a suitable relative or friend to ask, they could, in pairs and with permission, very politely approach the school secretary, caretaker, dinner assistant, school visitor or school governor for help. (Remind them to remember to say, 'Thank you very much for your time.')

When the questionnaires have been completed, individuals or pairs can prepare a short (five-minute) talk about a particular job, providing visual aids if possible (pictures of the uniform, photos, equipment and so on.)

Finally, ask the children what they have learned. Did they realize before how much is involved in having a job? Which jobs did they like the sound of? Will this influence them in

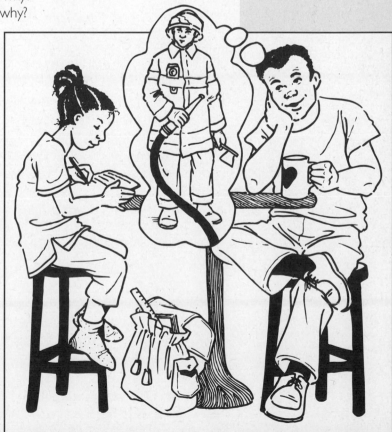

OBJECTIVES

To enable children to:
- focus on key skills relevant to learning and work
- gain understanding of the world of work
- interview adults, talk to adults and listen to adult experiences
- start to think about what types of job they might like in the future.

CROSS-CURRICULAR LINKS

ENGLISH

Exploring and developing ideas, insights and opinions; reporting and describing observations; listening and responding to a range of people; extended writing.

ICT

Using equipment for a variety of purposes, including word-processing.

the future? (They might be inspired to work harder to get the qualifications necessary for their favourite job!)

NOW OR LATER

■ The class could make an alphabet of jobs/careers to be put up on the wall and added to from time to time, for example:

A. astronaut, ambulance driver, architect…

B. baker, bank clerk, builder…

C. charity worker, cook…

■ Children could do a piece of extended writing about the job they would most like, perhaps describing 'A day in the life of…'

■ Children could consider the 'jobs' done by volunteers for various charities, and how some people choose to use their skills in helping others. Such voluntary workers could be interviewed along the same lines as for paid workers, and children could assess their overall contribution to society as well as finding out how many local groups are run by volunteers.

TEST SURVIVAL SKILLS

OBJECTIVES

To enable children to:
■ develop key skills relevant to learning and work
■ understand more about the way that tests and exams work
■ learn specific skills for test/ exam success
■ learn that it's OK to make mistakes, but learn from them.

CROSS-CURRICULAR LINKS

ENGLISH

Reading; understanding instructions; writing; sharing ideas, insights and opinions.

ICT

Using equipment for a variety of purposes.

RESOURCES AND CLASSROOM ORGANIZATION

You will need: a copy of photocopiable page 63, a sheet of paper and scissors for each child.

There is one activity for a pair/group, followed by a class discussion. Prepare in advance a 'fun' test which could be done on another day under exam conditions. This test should have examples of different ways of answering questions, such as filling in information in a given space, ticking/putting a cross in the right box, underlining/ringing the correct answer, and so on.

WHAT TO DO

Ask the children how they feel about the prospect of the many tests and exams they will be asked to do in the future, for example SATs. Most people admit to feeling anxious about being tested on anything – music, sports trials, tests for swimming certificates and so on. It is really helpful to know exactly what is expected by testers, and prepare for and practise similar tests in advance of the real thing. This goes for written tests in school as well.

Suggest that two children could actually know and understand exactly the same, but during a test, one could score higher marks than the other because of the way he or she did the test or exam. The person had a better 'exam technique'. Tell the children that this is what they are going to learn about next.

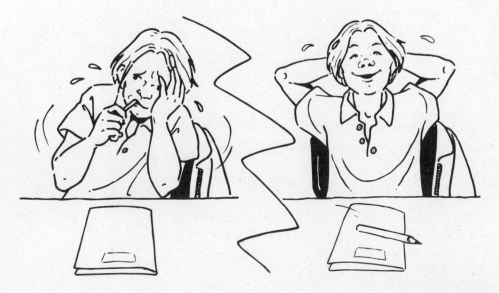

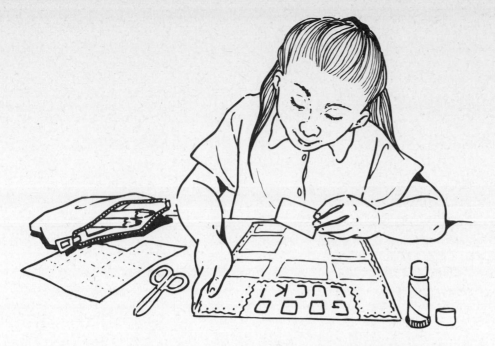

Give everyone a copy of photocopiable page 63 and explain that all the ideas on the sheet will help them with tests and exams. Explain that they are going to cut along the dotted lines on the sheet and discuss and sort out the 'tips' into three groups on the blank paper – those for 'A' *before* a test, 'B' *during* the test, and 'C' *near the end*, when they think they have finished!

Allow ten to fifteen minutes for this, then discuss as a class the points in each category. The children should then glue their slips of paper onto the blank paper under the headings 'Before', 'During' and 'Near the end' of the test.

Can the children think of any other good advice? For example, to check beforehand that they have a working pen, sharpened pencils, a ruler and so on, and not to stay up too late the previous evening.

Follow on now, or on another day, with your 'fun' test. Set up the classroom or hall as for a real test/exam – that is, with separate desks, a quiet place, a visible clock and so on. Explain to the children that they are going to do a practice 'fun' test, and remind them of the tips for working during the test and for when they think they have finished.

After the 15 minutes allowed, ask them to put their pens down. Tell them *they* are now going to be the 'examiners' and check how they have done. Read out the answers and/or explain how the answer should have been written to get a mark. Point out that even if the answer is technically right, if they have for example put a cross instead of a tick in a box, they have not answered correctly and must not give themselves a mark! Add that it is easy to make a mistake like this, but they can learn from it now so that they don't make the same mistake in a real exam or test. The exercise demonstrates the importance of reading the question carefully. Congratulate those with high marks and those who have tried hard.

Finally, ask the children whether they now feel more confident about tackling tests in the future. Reassure them that you will be giving them more help and explanations in plenty of time before each test, and anyone can ask for help.

> **Answers to 'Test survival skills' on photocopiable page 63**
>
> A: 4, 5, 9 and 12
> B: 1, 3, 6, 7, 8 and 10

NOW OR LATER

■ Challenge the children to make up their own simple tests and try them out on one another.

■ Let the children practise other types of tests or past papers under 'exam conditions'.

■ Children could produce their own checklist of exam tips under the three headings 'Before', 'During' and 'Near the end' of the exam/test. These could be printed out on a computer and mounted with a decorative border, or on a 'good luck' card. ('Good luck' can be helped by good preparation!)

Photocopiables

Name   Date

Self-assessment sheet

■ Tick the boxes that apply to you.

	Always/ every day	Usually/ regularly	Sometimes	Hardly ever
School work skills				
I listen attentively.				
I concentrate.				
I can work independently.				
I have a positive attitude to work.				
I can plan ahead.				
I am able to learn from my mistakes.				
I do my homework carefully.				
I finish my work.				
I am happy to try new things.				
I do my best.				
Group and teamwork skills				
I co-operate with others.				
I contribute to group work.				
I am a good member of a team.				
Behaviour				
I am polite.				
I am thoughtful.				
I am sensible.				
I am helpful.				
Personal				
I can reflect on my own experiences.				
I am well organized.				
I make healthy choices.				
I am careful about safety.				
I take exercise.				
I am trustworthy.				
I am responsible.				
Relationships				
I respect differences in people.				
I show concern for others.				
I am a good friend.				
I am pleased to meet new people.				
Society/citizenship				
I look after other people's possessions.				
I look after school property.				
I am a good member of my school community.				
I care for my local environment.				

I am especially proud of _____.

I would like to improve _____.

Signed: _____ Teacher's signature: _____

Class/Year: _____   School: _____

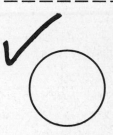

Test survival skills

■　Cut along the dotted lines and sort the tips into these three categories:

Before the test/exam.

Working **during** the exam.

Near the end, when you think you've finished!

---

1. Watch the time carefully. Don't spend too long on one question.

2. Make sure you haven't missed any pages or questions!

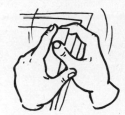

3. Read instructions carefully, for example how many questions to do.

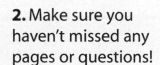

4. Be sure that you know when each test/exam is being held, so you have plenty of time to revise.

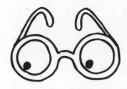

5. Do some practice tests or old exam papers if possible.

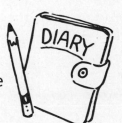

6. If you can't do a question, don't panic. Leave it until the end, and go back and try again.

---

7. Check how much information is needed in your answer. For example, if two marks are available, you probably need to make two points.

8. Look carefully to see how to answer the question, for example you might have to tick a box or put a ring around the right answer.

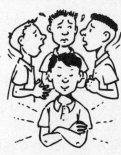

9. On the day of the test/exam, keep calm. Don't "wind up" your friends by saying how nervous you are or how you don't know anything.

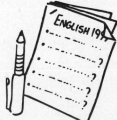

10. Read the question really slowly and carefully first.

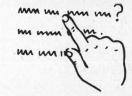

11. Read though your answers to check that they make sense and to see if you remember anything extra.

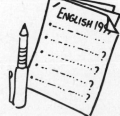

12. When revising, don't just read through your work but *test* yourself, or ask someone else to test you by asking you questions. Don't leave it until the night before the exam!

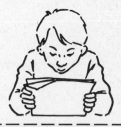

NATIONAL STANDARDS FOR KEY SKILLS

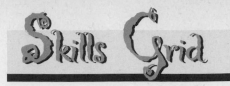

The grid below will help you to identify which activities can be used to develop specific key skills, and enable you to check on the overall balance of skill development in your teaching programme. These skills are based on the QCA's *National Standards for Key Skills.*

SKILLS DEVELOPED IN SECTIONS:	1	2	3	4	5	6	7	8
				IN ACTIVITIES:				
Improving own learning and performance	1–5	1–6	1–3	1–5	1–3	1–4	1–3	1–3
Communication	1–5	1–5	1–3	1–5	1–3	1–4	1–3	1–3
Problem-solving	1, 4	1–3, 6	1–3	1–4	___	1–3	1	3
Working with others	1–3	1–4	1–3	1–3, 5	1–4	1–4	1–3	2, 3
Practical skills	5	3, 5, 6	1	1	___	2	2	2, 3